From Wits' End to John O'Groats

A Journey by Les Roberts

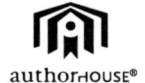

AuthorHouse™ UK Ltd.
500 Avebury Boulevard
Central Milton Keynes, MK9 2BE
www.authorhouse.co.uk
Phone: 08001974150

© 2009 Les Roberts. All rights reserved.

No part of this book may be reproduced, stored in a retrieval system, or transmitted by any means without the written permission of the author.

First published by AuthorHouse 8/3/2009

ISBN: 978-1-4389-6835-3 (sc)

This book is printed on acid-free paper.

Thanks to :

Hannah: for love, tea, typing and tolerance.
Mark Stewart-Jones: for his encouragement, endless advice and moral support.
Tom Isaacs and everyone at the Cure Parkinson's Trust - Movers & Shakers: whose message and example inspired me to do this.
Peter Fletcher: for rescuing the mission when one of the support drivers withdrew at the last minute.
The rest of the squad: for being such a supportive and amiable bunch.

And those chums: who, throughout my sporting life, have been there and made the difference.

Foreword

When you have Parkinson's for 16 years it is impossible to ride one thousand miles in just 12 days. Les Roberts thrives on mission impossible.

This book tells of a quiet, unassuming man and how he achieved the unachievable. Marvel at his modesty, relish his turn of phrase (and pace) but above all be inspired by his inner strength and resilience in the face of the biggest challenge of his life.

It is through the extraordinary feats (and feet) of Les and people like him that we too can achieve our goal and cure the hitherto incurable.

Tom Isaacs
Co-Founder, President of The Cure Parkinson's Trust and Mover & Shaker

A Journey within a Journey

What is it about an extreme that makes it so fascinating? Beginnings, ends, firsts, lasts, mosts, leasts all seem to generate intrigue and attract special status even when the subject, in all other respects, is barely worthy of note.

So it is with the two places that are furthest away from each other on the British mainland. In the far southwest, Land's End is undeniably a dramatic stretch of coastline but it is not outstanding. I would be surprised if there are not many other equally, if not more, impressive locations to be found even within Cornwall. At the northern extremity lies John O'Groats, which, if I describe it as *a loose cluster of buildings in the top right hand corner of Caithness*, I might still be accused of "larging it up". Yet, because of where they are situated, both these places enjoy broad recognition and acclaim.

But there is no such ambivalence about the journey that links them. Its celebrity status as a classic challenge for the self-propelled is wholly justified and the popularity of LeJOG, as the trip is affectionately known, remains undiminished.

For Ian Bashford, a member of the Old Portlians Cycling Club in southeast London, riding end to end, had been an ambition for years and so, as soon as he had served his time in the Met. Police, amongst the first things to go onto his post retirement agenda was fulfilling this wish. It took him the best part of a year to pull it all together – establishing a route, booking accommodation, arranging transport and support services and assembling a group of like-minded, and compatible individuals with whom he could share the adventure.

I didn't come into the picture until very late in the day. I was looking for a platform on which to raise funds for The Cure Parkinson's Trust (CPT) and Ian's plan sounded the sort of thing I had in mind. I approached him about a place on the ride and his agreement was as magnanimous as it was immediate: I say "magnanimous" because on the face of it, although an experienced cyclist of many years' standing (perhaps that should be pedaling) I was not particularly fit and, being a person with Parkinson's, there was considerable potential for me to be a liability to him and the rest of the team.

Even some of my nearest and dearest friends, who had accompanied me on many a successful sporting mission over the years couldn't disguise their scepticism about what I was proposing to do. Should a 64 year old 16 years after being diagnosed with Parkinson's really be thinking about riding a bike over 1000 miles in 12 consecutive days?

I really didn't know whether I was being courageous, foolhardy, irresponsible or what. I had been riding fairly regularly over the previous few years but whether I was up to something as stern as this was another matter. Perhaps self delusion is a symptom of PD but I simply reckoned that, as long as my hard wiring[1] was still intact, I should

---
[1] Hard wiring refers to the motor-skills and mental processes that I developed and practiced with such intensity over so many years that they became intuitive and spontaneous

be able to ride myself in and give a reasonable account of myself; a strategy that had always worked in the past.

Only after I had publicly committed myself to the ride and started to attract sponsorship money, did the enormity of it all begin to sink in. I could no longer rely on any residual fitness and the amount and quality of the riding I had managed to do in the previous 12 months was scarcely adequate preparation for a ride that would have been a challenge even in the days when being athletically fit was taken for granted. On top of that there was all the uncertainty associated with my Parkinson's – how would it manifest itself, would my medication maintain its effectiveness under such prolonged duress and would the periodic dystonia[2] in my left biceps and shoulder cause me problems when pulling on or even just holding my handlebars? This had been a regular source of discomfort even on rides half the length of the average daily mileage planned for LeJOG.

It really wasn't looking such a clever idea any more. However, I clung onto the thought that there would always be the option of climbing into the sag wagon[3] if ever or, as seemed more likely, whenever things got too much for me and it was this failsafe that finally persuaded me to go for it.

The hard wiring I referred to must have germinated in the mid to late 1950s when I was a pupil at the Roan

---
[2] Dystonia is a neurological movement disorder characterized by involuntary muscle contractions, which force certain parts of the body into abnormal, sometimes painful, movements or postures.
[3] Sag wagon. A cycling term for a support/rescue vehicle

Grammar School in Greenwich. I always seemed to be one of the first home in the obligatory training runs and inter-house cross country matches up and down the hills of Greenwich Park and this invariably led to my being called upon to represent the school. I found little to enjoy; I vividly recall that taste of blood as the cold air scoured my lungs and airways. Just as the summers back then seemed to be endless sunshine so cross-country running always seemed to take place on raw, grey afternoons.

But my pride wouldn't allow me to coast round and, what's more, it was an opportunity to get one over on the big kids, which meant nearly everyone else, because I was a tiny youth standing 1.30m (4ft 3ins) and weighing 26kgs (just over 4 stones) when I was 12. I suppose it was at this time that I first came to realize that athletic competition and pain were pretty much synonymous.

I got involved with racing bikes when I was 14. I joined a local club and cut my teeth going out on their Sunday runs, which would include rides out to local race circuits to watch the Club's teams competing against the best of the other clubs in the region. I found it enthralling; the bright colours, the expensive Italian and French bikes and equipment, the distinctive 'ping' of rock hard tubular racing tyres on tarmac and the evocative aroma of horse liniment. This was for me: I was hooked.

By the time I was 19 I had outgrown several bikes and built up one of those exotic, Italian equipped lightweight machines. Most Sundays I could be found riding it at one race circuit or another representing the West Kent

Road Club whose bright orange and blue vest I wore with pride. I raced through the 1960s and into the early 70s achieving first category status in my first year as a senior, and maintaining it throughout my racing career, which took me to 2 other clubs, the Airedale Olympic CRC in 1969 and the CC Basingstoke in 1973. I would regularly ride around 200-300 miles a week of which 60 – 120 would be racing.

I shot up in height very quickly during my teens – 45cm in 4 years – although I didn't get much wider. I remained very slight, which meant I was never able to develop enough brute force to compete with the roadman sprinters who tended to dominate the shorter, faster races. My tally of winning rides therefore remained relatively modest although I was always up there, in the thick of things, rarely finishing outside the top 10 and frequently in the top 6. My particular strengths emerged in the hills and whenever attrition was the name of the game. The more climbing that had to be done and the tougher the conditions the more I came into my own.

My dream initially was to take the sport all the way and turn professional but once I started mixing it with the big guns at national level it became clear this would be a desperately hard way to earn a crust.

Then, in 1974, I made a move that spelt the beginning of the end for bike racing: I bought a house. At first, the essential works required on the place had to be fitted in and around my day job and training schedule but it soon became evident that attempting to do all three would result in my not doing justice to any of them. Something had to go and at this stage in my life it had to be the bike. By 1975 my trusty steed had been decommissioned and found a new home in the back of the garage.

Three years of DIY and turbo-charged socializing later, I felt I'd had a surfeit of both activities and I wanted more shape and discipline in my life; I needed to get back into sport. By this time bicycles had lost much of their allure but destiny was about to pull a masterstroke

Whilst waiting for an old school friend in his squash club I overheard a conversation between two lads sitting close by. One was telling his mate how his recent good form was down to a fitness regime devised for him by his brother who had some connection with the famous athletics club, the Blackheath Harriers. He went on to say that he had been surprised to discover that the club wasn't based anywhere near Blackheath but in Hayes, Kent. He wasn't the only one for whom this was news.

I have never seen either of the two conversationalists since nor have I ever discovered who the brother might have been but just catching those few words was to prove one of the seminal moments of my life: maybe *the* seminal moment.

Hayes was no distance from where I lived and so, one evening, towel, shorts and dodgy plimsolls in hand and the promise I had shown at school in mind, I ventured through the hallowed portals of that esteemed athletics institution - and suffered one of the greatest hidings of my life. Four miles of local trails, courtesy of a couple of the club's veteran athletes, had me groveling and gasping. And if that wasn't humbling enough, I later learnt they were both way past their best and one of them wasn't even a runner but a javelin thrower. I had grossly underestimated the standard of club-level running.

Despite that rude awakening and the further bashings I took in those early days I stuck at it and, driven by determination and a doggedness, which I can only imagine came from my cycle racing days, I very quickly found myself an integral part of the senior track and field squad for the 5,000m, 10,000m and the 3,000m steeplechase At this time Blackheath Harriers were going through a purple patch as they rose from the Southern League to the top division of the British League in 4 consecutive seasons as champions each year. It was a particularly exhilarating and rewarding time to be a "'Heathen."

Come the 1984 track season I had turned 40 and been designated a "Veteran" (subsequently renamed "Master") but I certainly had no intention of taking this as a cue to slow down: far from it. I could still be relied upon to run well inside 15 minutes for 5,000m and sub 31 minutes for 10,000m, which meant I remained very much part of the Harriers' firepower.

In fact, given the level of competition to which I was then being regularly exposed, I was still learning and improving and it was perhaps not surprising that I should shine brightly when competing solely against my peers.

That year I won the European Masters 5,000m track title and took silver in the 10,000m with silver again in the 10k Road Championship held in Berne. Then, in 1985, in the Olympic Stadium in Rome, I managed to produce a final lap of 60 seconds flat to win the World Masters 5,000m Championship. I continued to improve through 1986 and was rewarded with a number of invitations to take part in the lucrative masters road-racing scene in the US. This didn't make me a rich man though: there were far too many distractions. But I did make enough to have a hell of a good time and come out even.

Throughout my running career my trump card was my sprint finish. With about 150m to go I could come off virtually any pace and accelerate to the line. Even if I was at my wits' end entering the last lap of a 5,000m or 10,000m race I could still produce it. It was a tremendous asset that brought me many victories even when I had looked (and felt) out of the running.

I have likened it to pulling the lever on an aircraft ejector seat - total, once-and-for-all commitment. There was no room for hesitation or tactics. Everything that wasn't essential for running as fast as possible was shut down; this meant all pain and anxiety was suppressed and replaced by a sense of soaring. It was as if I entered a different dimension.

I have no recall of the finish of any of my races involving a sprint to the line and I never once saw who followed me in because I was too busy dealing with the nausea that always overwhelmed me as I eased up after the line. This was the result of blood flooding back into the various organs, especially my stomach, from where it had been borrowed by my legs and the other bits crucial for running flat out. I was not a pretty sight immediately post race by all accounts. I've always thought it odd that I should have had this turn of speed when competing on foot yet it had been my principal weakness on the bike.

I peaked in 1987 and 1988, two years in which I rarely failed to either win my event or post a personal best time. During this time I had a win in the B string 5,000m in the British League, set an age related world record for the 1-hour run of 18,555m (11.5 miles) and was top of the UK Master's ranking lists at both 5,000m and 10,000m for the 4 years 1985–1988 (ranked 60th at 10,000m nationally in absolute terms). Come 1989, although I continued to run reasonably well, it was patchy and I struggled to find the consistent sharpness of the preceding years.

Then early in 1990 the first in a series of events took place, which were as unexpected as they were life-changing.

In the March I found myself on the rough end of a broken relationship that left me extremely low. My reaction to this angst was to become immersed in my work, which left little time for running. I did, however, maintain contact with the Club and at the end of October, by way of a change of scenery as much as anything, I linked up with a Blackheath team who were traveling down to the south of France to run the Marseilles to Cassis Semi-Marathon. This international classic regularly attracted over 10,000 participants and I had won the Masters division of the race in both 1987 and 1988 and was then still the Masters' course record holder (66m.33s). My plan was to watch the race from the sidelines or, better still, hitch a ride in one of the official cars. I had not run a step for 8 months so there was no reason to take any running kit with me.

When we got there, however, a powerful combination of the intoxicating atmosphere and a number of influential, persuasive tongues meant I found myself standing on the start line amongst the elite competitors wearing a borrowed vest and shorts and a pair of racing shoes hastily acquired from a local retailer - feeling a complete sham. As nice as it is to be acknowledged and appreciated, especially far from home, on this occasion I really could have done without the well-wishers who came up to say hello and encourage me in Gallic tones to "make a good race" or called me "Less" from behind the spectator barrier and then inclined an arm upwards with a snake-like motion, presumably depicting the "Col de la Gineste" (the mountain that constitutes the first half of the race) whilst indicating the number 1 to suggest they were expecting me to win again: how embarrassing.

I desperately wanted to explain my position to them all and apologise in advance for disappointing them. But, as it was, all I could do was grin and bear it and pray for the race to get under way so that I could disappear into the maelstrom of slaver and elbows that is the first mile or so of any mass participation event. (There's always that bunch of bozos who barge through to the front in an attempt to get their faces in the local papers only to melt into the tarmac and obscurity again just up the road.)

The cannon employed to start this race every year doesn't just sound off it punches your lights out from the inside, but I welcomed the sensation as it heralded escape from my far greater discomfort standing on the start line.

It took a lot of self-discipline and concentration to get through that race respectably. It was not much fun because in order to remain focused on running the shortest line as smoothly and economically as possible it was necessary to blank out everything else - the other runners, the gradient, the scenery. It was like running down a narrow corridor for 13 miles. I finished 105th in 72m.30s and remember feeling disappointed that I had just failed to make the top 1%. But it was short lived and elation soon took over. Although over 7 minutes down on the time I would have expected if trained up, in terms of sheer application and making something out of nothing it was arguably one of my best ever athletic performances. It certainly demonstrated that my fitness decay rate must have been very slow and provided a perfect example of "hard wiring" at work.

You would think this performance would have inspired me to start training again but it didn't. My emotions were still in tatters and I continued to bury myself in my work. In the spring of 1991 I started studying at the London School of Sports Massage to become a sports massage therapist. The course was extremely absorbing but even adding this further diversion to the demands of my day job still didn't provide me with sufficient distraction to overcome my bleakness.

I qualified at the end of 1991 and almost immediately found myself swamped with requests for help. There weren't many massage therapists about in those days so I was soon in the pleasing position of being able to give something back to the sports that had given so much to me. In the event, however, the work was so gratifying that it felt like I was still taking rather than giving anything back. My debt seemed destined to grow and grow.

I was invited to go to the world cross - country championships in Boston, USA in March 1992 as part of the medical back up to the Great Britain cross-country squad. It was a priceless experience if a little daunting when I realised the professional status of the bodies I would quite literally have in the palms of my hands.

On the face of it life was rich and varied but still I couldn't shake off the feelings of desolation that cast a shadow over everything I did. It had to be something more profound than the lingering heartache of a lost love so it was time to unload my woe onto my GP, poor chap, to see what he made of it all. He diagnosed clinical depression, put me on vitamins and referred me on to a specialist who in turn said there wasn't a great deal he could do for me as I had already analysed, rationalised and every other "ised" my own situation very thoroughly. Nevertheless he conceded that a few sessions with a therapist might help but there was a waiting list of 48 weeks!

He gave me the number of someone I could approach privately and on my first visit a few days later I found myself standing outside a drab, mock Tudor pile on the outskirts of Bromley. Going inside was like stepping into a Dickensian novel. The place was crammed with heavy, dark wood furniture and smelt musty. It was also dimly lit and decidedly chilly; hardly the ideal conditions for encouraging people to bare their souls and voice their problems and anxieties. My first meeting with the therapist did little to assuage my misgivings; a shabby, weasely, little man, who blended so effectively into his dingy, antiquated surroundings that it was easy to lose track of him when he wasn't moving about and raising dust.

After a couple of totally unenlightening one-to-one sessions he suggested that I would benefit from joining a therapy group. I agreed but was somewhat taken aback by having to commit myself to sessions for weeks at a time. I was even more dismayed to discover during the first of these gatherings that the majority of those in the group had been going for years and there seemed to be an assumption that I would be joining them. I stuck it out for a couple of weeks but rapidly came to the conclusion that this wasn't for me; it was making me depressed! The others in the group had difficulties far more entrenched than mine; they seemed individually and collectively institutionalized, programmed to perpetuate their condition, determined to find a negative side to everything and to identify with it. I doubted these sessions would lead to answers to the problems being presented but, dare I say it, it occurred to me that perhaps it wasn't in anyone's interest to find any.

I continued to run recreationally from time to time but it all seemed very different. It was as if I was running across an incline or on a steep camber all the time. My stride was uneven and it was pointed out to me on more than one occasion that my left arm wasn't swinging: it felt normal to me. I had also developed a very slight limp when walking and would experience tremulousness whenever confronted by anything even vaguely unfamiliar or stressful like making a formal phone call. The year before, despite feeling very confident, I'd had great difficulty controlling my nerves and keeping my handwriting legible when I sat my massage therapy exams. The examiner had been moved to remark that mine was probably the untidiest paper he had ever had the misfortune to have to wade through. That didn't sound at all like me. At the time I put it down to the fact that they were my first written exams for 30 years.

Towards the end of 1992 I took some advanced anatomy and physiology modules as part of my ongoing massage studies and in the course of my reading around the subjects I came across descriptions of some common neurological conditions. It was chilling reading; I could tick so many of the boxes. After my previous experience of trying to see a specialist on the NHS I went straight to a local private hospital and bought £90–worth of a consultant neurologist's time, which would be mine within the week. When the time came, it took the consultant no more than a couple of minutes, feeling each joint in turn while I waved around its opposite number, for him to make his diagnosis. "There is no easy way to say this," he said almost apologetically – "you have got Parkinson's Disease."

When my ears had stopped ringing from that bombshell, I found myself sitting on the wall outside the hospital not horrified and despairing as you might expect but almost relieved that there was an explanation for what had been happening to me. More significant, though, was the realisation that my black shadow had gone. This was relief beyond words and I can honestly say I felt more positive about things at that moment than at any time during the previous 3 years. Being told I had Parkinson's obviously wasn't exactly good news but, crucially, it looked like I had been given back the wherewithal to deal with it or at least give it a good run for its money.

A second appointment with the consultant was scheduled for the following week but this time in his NHS clinic at Bromley Hospital. He explained the condition more thoroughly and reassured me about its likely progress, available drugs, etc. I also learned that my depressive state could well have been the leading edge of the Parkinson's although why it should have lifted with the diagnosis remained a mystery to me. (I would discover in time that my newly acquired condition was both quirky and bespoke and anomalies were commonplace.)

Before I left I was introduced to the specialist nurse, Jane, a stunning young lady who, judging by my own reaction on meeting her, must have triggered more involuntary movement amongst her male patients than she ever prevented. I was told she was always contactable should I need advice or help with anything. There followed a few moments of wishful thinking.

Outside the clinic it really did feel as if this was the first day of the rest of my life. How things unfolded from that point on would depend on my ability to recognize and manage the Parkinson's. I decided to walk the 3 miles home; not a major act of defiance but a nod in the right direction, I thought. On the way I rehearsed how and to whom I should relate my news and a mantra emerged, which more or less summed up how I felt –

"If this thing insists on moving in with me then it's going to be on my bloody terms"

Over the next 16 years I endeavored to uphold that declaration and was helped immeasurably by being allowed to phase out my involvement at work, going part-time in the spring of 1993 and retiring altogether in 1996. These arrangements had been given the nod quite some time before my PD was diagnosed. My original idea was to set up in business as a massage therapist and then go off traveling round the world to weird and wonderful places participating in novel races from time to time like the Marathon des Sables 6-day endurance race across the Sahara and the Everest Marathon in Nepal. In the event, of course, I had to set aside these grand aspirations but I went ahead with the retirement plan as it afforded me the privilege of being able to control more or less all demands made on me. Such a relatively stress-free existence would prove a godsend for living with Parkinson's.

I continued my association with the Blackheath Harriers through the 90s and took over the administration of the club's social activities. I had ideas about running again but they were soon dashed when I found I had become very injury prone, probably as a result of my now suspect reflexes and unreliable proprioception[4]. At the best of times it doesn't take much to crock a runner.

But I wasn't to be denied participation in sport. Through another timely piece of synchronicity I was introduced to field archery. This grabbed me in the way only bike racing and running had ever done before and had me driving up and down the land most weekends to compete. I loved it and it was good that I should be exercising my upper body for a change. Sadly the group I teamed up with gave up the sport after a couple of years, which led to my drifting away from it as well.

With the passing of my mum in August 1999 and not having any competitive sport to train for, the time was ripe to do some long haul traveling. At various times over the next few years I went to Syria, Cuba, Namibia, USA, Australia, Hong Kong, Singapore, New Zealand and Egypt. At first I found globetrotting fairly taxing especially negotiating airports but I learned to pace myself

---

[4] Proprioceptors provide information about muscle tension and the position of our joints and are central to the body's equilibrium

and always to allow plenty of time for things. Pressure and Parkinson's just do not make happy bedfellows.

Cycling also started to feature again and an annual trip to see close up a couple of stages of the Tour de France – usually in the Alps – became established as one of the highlights of each summer. Other rides included a 10 day 550 mile Millennium tour round the East Cape of New Zealand, which ended up in the city of Gisborne where we were amongst the first people on the planet to see the sun come up on 1.1.2000. And in 2007 the target was a 108-mile, single day ride from Dieppe to Paris in aid of the Parkinson's Appeal. We did it in a bit under 7 hours and that result opened the way for me to undertake much longer rides than I had previously thought possible. It also gave me the justification to treat myself to a new state-of-the-art "dream machine" road bike (see appendix 1).

Then in the summer of 2008, my 16 year-old proclamation was set its stiffest test yet as I joined the Old Portlians in their assault on   LeJOG.

"Cometh the hour..."

The Cast

Ian "Bashers" Bashford – captain and chief engineer.

Dave "Dangerous" Hickman – principal stabilizing force.

Barry "Disco" Meens – archivist and international gastronomy consultant.

Jerry "Jezzer" Hancock – security *ubermeister* and leading windbreak.

John "Father Jack" Mulvaney – head of culture and classics with special responsibility for acrobatic display.

Dave "Oz" Osborn – chief cynic & dispenser of *bons mots*.

Steve "Paper Boy" Lennell – professor of transport and logistics.

Peter Fletcher – variously referred to as "Saviour" and "God" – MD of everything else.

Me – (As far as I know I didn't have a pseudonym) - privileged guest and witness.

The Route

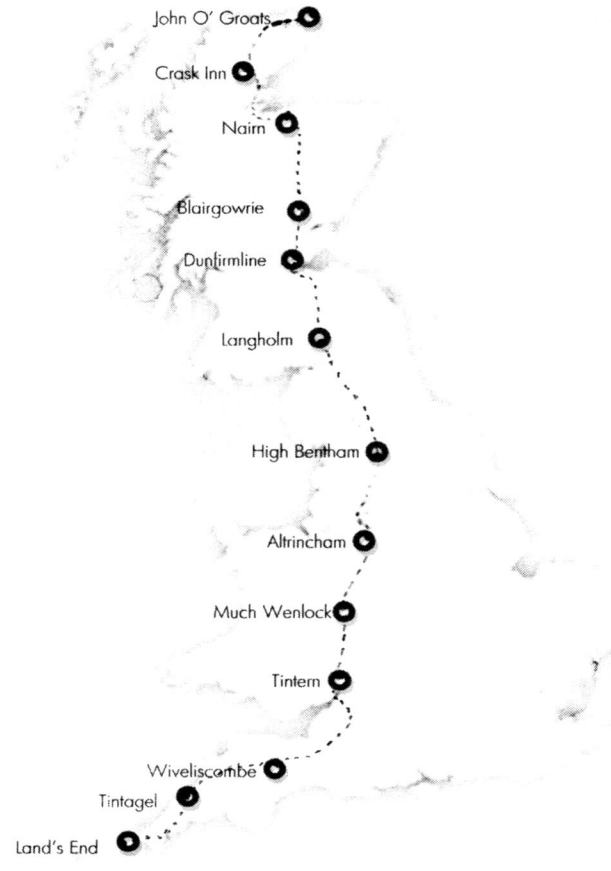

Sunday 15th June

Go West Old Man.

At 9 o'clock sharp, a white minibus bursting at the seams with bikes and bike riders made its way out of the car park of Blackheath and Bromley Harriers Athletics Club in Hayes, Kent, en route to Land's End, Cornwall. This was the Old Portlians Cycling Club's expeditionary force, which was making its way to the start of a 12-day bike-riding odyssey.

Its destination was reached by early evening everything having gone remarkably smoothly. Nevertheless, 9 hours cooped up in a glorified Transit van with 8 bikes and enough tools, spare parts and baggage to open a medium size shop was a long time for highly-tuned athletic specimens like us. Having tumbled and fallen out of the bus like so many bags of soiled laundry most of us faced the daunting task of straightening limbs, un-cricking necks, un-numbing bums and coaxing contorted torsos back into something resembling humanoid form, (a particularly futile exercise for those whose posture was quasimodal at the best of times).

Once unfurled, we set about unloading the bus; there was certainly a lot of stuff.

"Ee, best be safe than sorry, eh, me oud love?" as they might say in Arkengarsidethwaitesbottomroydsgillbeck, (which I'm sure we ride through on stage 6)

After a period of concentrated bike assembling and maintenance and sorting out rooming arrangements for the night, the next thing on the agenda was to locate an establishment that could satisfy our pressing need for food. The Old Success Inn in Sennen Cove was strongly recommended as a very good place to eat, which was just as well because as far as we could tell it was the only place. We found it nestling at the bottom of a lane that was so precipitous it was difficult to walk down, especially for poor old Oz who was still feeling the effects of a recent hip operation and the bus ride. Someone said: "I hope there's not going to be too many climbs like that on our route." Some hope.

The First Of Many?
The bar menu met with everyone's approval and the local ale slipped down nicely. Spirits were high, laughter abounded and any misgivings about what we were about to attempt over the next 12 days were temporarily shelved. The mixture of our garrulousness and the striking black and red commemorative polo shirts that most of the lads were sporting could easily have given the impression that

we were a touring rugby club, although what position in the team anyone would think I commanded with my 57 kilo frame is hard to imagine. One young couple took interest in the commotion we were causing and kindly donated £20 when they heard about the CPT and what we were attempting to do. This was the first of many such gestures that we would encounter during the course of our journey. Although everyone was looking forward to hitting the road the next morning, there was no disguising the fact that each of us was harbouring at least a little anxiety about the challenge that lay ahead. Most of us seemed to be suffering some sort of dysfunction or discomfort. Bashers had major back surgery scheduled for after the ride; Oz wasn't out of the woods yet with his hip and Dangerous Dave's wellness was prone to compromise as a result of his tendency to work too long and hard. As for me, I now had an inflamed elbow to contend with on top of my usual basket of Parkinsonian foibles. Only Jezzer seemed immune to the ravages of wear and tear but then he is moulded out of airstrip quality concrete and in any case at 39 is only a babe compared to the rest of us.

Transcript from audio-log
Back at the B&B now and I am feeling decidedly stuffed. A chalkboard behind the bar had listed some irresistible desserts and I lost no time justifying my need for one; the treacle sponge with treacle sauce was essential for topping up my carbohydrate reserves. The dense sponge, the size of a large orange, came in a sea of glutinous, dark brown ooze: sensational! They say that cyclists burn up to 150 calories every 15 minutes. Given the muscle tension and involuntary

movements associated with Parkinson's, my fuel consumption can probably match that when I'm free-wheeling down hill with the wind behind me.

Peter has now turned up and seems a tad unsteady on his feet having gone into the bar downstairs for a nightcap, or three. He thinks the Dictaphone that I'm using is a phone and he wants to make a witty contribution, as inebriates are wont to do. All the signs are that he'll not be awake for long. I shall just watch a bit of telly then it will be shut-eye for me too. Early night. It's about 10pm.

Monday 16th June

Land's End to Tintagel (Cornwall)
Mileage 89m
Ascent 7000ft

Transcript cont.
My watch is beeping urgently. It is 6.15 am and a consignment of undiluted sunshine is being delivered through the window and is expediting my rise into consciousness; a perfect awakening on what looks like a perfect day for a spin on a bicycle with chums. Let's hope Bashers ordered 12 of these.

Several times during the night Peter attempted to get into the wardrobe before eventually locating the bathroom. I'm so glad his radar had only developed a delay and hadn't failed altogether. He is now awake and is absolutely fine. He thinks that he had an early, undisturbed night. Of course he did.

Following the exchange of farewells with our amiable hosts, we made our way down to the coastline for the obligatory photo-shoot. Enthusiasm was high but it wasn't long before indecision and confusion set in as to who was going to take a picture of whom and against what background. However, salvation was at hand, arriving amidst a cloud of smoke, a squeal of tyres and with a cry of, "give me 5 minutes." It was the official photographer who privately operated a photoset, complete with signpost to John O'Groats. For a fee he took a couple of pictures with a sensible camera before allowing us the freedom of his facility to take snaps of our own.

Gimme Shelter

The first pedal revolution of our thousand-mile trip was made in brilliant sunshine. This was a great start but once on the open road it soon became evident that we were ploughing into a stiff headwind. How could this be? Rides from Land's End to John O'Groats are always accompanied by favourable southwesterly tail winds, aren't they? The permanent orientation of the braced hunch adopted by every tree and bush as far as the eye could see bore witness to this. It was in the rules of engagement! Be that as it may, there was no getting away from it, we were in for a tough opening stage. Bashers and Jezzer were, predictably, the strong men and took the lead for most of the way, which afforded the rest of us some shelter. As I was feeling a bit dysfunctional, I was pleased to be able to ride at the very back of the group where I was able to take maximum advantage of the shielding on offer. My elbow was giving me grief as I struggled to hang on but I persevered and was relieved to find that, even though I was being put through the mangle, I was still keeping up and by lunch was beginning to feel more comfortable. However, all the efforts of the morning, trying to overcome the bradykinesia (taught, sluggish muscles) affecting my left leg and arm meant that with 20 miles still to do I had "blown up" - depleted all my energy reserves - and could only watch as the others rode away leaving me to finish the day's ride at my own, more sedate pace. I ended up only a few minutes down on them, which, after 84 hilly miles, represented an extremely encouraging first day.

Bastard Hill

Our lunch stop had been in a little wayside pub just north of Truro. We relished the food when it came as it was hard earned. Four of the squad had somehow got snarled up in traffic on the way through Truro leaving three of us unexpectedly some way ahead. We decided we should stop and wait for the four and, as a lunch break was about due, we pulled into the pub we just happened to be passing. We then got a call from one of the lads behind who informed us we had gone the wrong way (God bless the mobile phone!). Democracy dictated that we retrace and join the others on the official route. This took us along a lane, not much better than a cart track, to a tiny hamlet called Idless where the crazed surface reared up into a slippery, back-wrenching 1 in 5 (20%) climb. Idless could not have been more aptly named. Id = "provenance", less = "without" ergo "without provenance" = "bastard." (Well, that's what I wanted to believe). You can imagine the exasperation of the three of us who had had to turn back, when, on reaching the top of the hill, we found ourselves face to face with the pub where we had been in the first place. Bugger Idless and a pox on the CTC[5] and its confounded route finders!

Sweet Dream

The first thing I saw on entering the pub made the despair that was Idless vanish instantly. There, writ large on the bar menu, was "suet pudding with treacle." Sadly there

---
[5] Cyclists Touring Club

wasn't any left. A couple of portions of that would have set me up for the rest of the trip. With the onset of universal concern with diet, this gem of an "after-pud" has seemingly, become almost extinct. I had to settle for lemon flan and ice cream, which was disappointingly lightweight and simply not in the same league at all. Energy and enthusiasm restored, we continued more or less in a northeasterly direction through Fiddlers Green, St. Newlyn East, St. Kew and Pendogett – wonderful names as undulating as the landscape they evoked – and on to our overnight stop at Tintagel where our final resting place for the day lay at the very top of the town: just what our legs needed!

The Most Important Meal

The lodgings in Tintagel were comfortable enough. The proprietor, though, was a miserable bugger who showed little sympathy for cyclists. We had to leave the bikes in the open where they were not particularly secure given their value. Contentment was restored at breakfast by the availability of a comprehensive and plentiful selection for what would, obviously, be a key meal for us each day. I was able to eat far more sensibly than the day before when I put myself outside a full English fry-up in the absence of much alternative; clearly a daft move for a fully paid up "mover and shaker."[6] Subsequently, I paid due regard to the constraints[7] of my medication and kept away from protein until evening and felt better for it.

---

[6] A person with Parkinson's.
[7] L.Dopa, my principal drug, is a synthetic protein, which means it can become overwhelmed in the presence of other protein and lose its potency

Tuesday 17th June

Tintagel (Cornwall) to Wiveliscombe (Somerset.) Mileage 87m Ascent 7780ft

Cornwall's Departing Gift

We managed to be on the road by 9:30 and, hallelujah, the southwesterlies had resumed prevailing. We headed off up the coast and everything looked good: gears whirred, tyres sang, hearts were uplifted and the cry went up, "Come on Devon, show us what you've got!" Unfortunately we had overlooked the possibility that Cornwall might not have finished with us yet. Kernow's departing gesture will be forever etched not only on my mind but also on the lining of my lungs. We had been coping well with a beautiful, but seriously rolling coast road when the ambush occurred. After voraciously consuming single hump undulations, we were suddenly hit by two multi-stage 1 in 5s (20%) in quick succession. They concentrated the mind but we were all up to the challenge and the two climbs were soon behind us and we had moved on to contemplating what delight Crackington Haven, the next place on our route, would bring. Crackington Haven is an ancient Cornish port apparently once favoured by Thomas Hardy and his Missus for days out. It had also been the setting for scenes in the TV series Poldark. It sounded worth a visit.

The lane leading down to it was narrow and unkempt and seemed to get narrower and more agricultural by the yard. At the same time the gradient increased from "steep" through "very steep" to "dodgy" then, finally, into the most extreme category, "oh shit!" At the bottom, seven ashen-faced bike riders, pulses racing, sphincters clenched, careered through the tiny port and found themselves immediately climbing back out again having almost literally paid the place a flying visit. The exit lane that rose from the seafront had, thankfully, acted as an emergency escape road but it then coiled back on itself and revealed its true colours.

Standing between us and the world outside, proudly displaying its status for all to see, was what could only be described as a barrier of mud, grass and tarmac – the "Great Wall of Crackington" - the identical twin of the bowel-loosening descent that we had plummeted down just moments before.

Four of the lads, Dave, Oz, Ian and John incredibly made it over this monster and Jezzer would have done so too if he hadn't chosen the inside line which looked more like a 1 in 2 (50%)! I had to take my hat off to them. I took the photo of the road sign and used that as an excuse to walk the really stiff bit. I would have needed a considerably smaller bottom gear than my 34x26 to conquer this one. We had known the day's route was going to be lumpy but nothing had prepared us for climbing of this order. In the first 15 miles we'd negotiated any number of hills between 8 and 12%, two at 20% and one at 30% and each one was preceded or followed by a comparable descent. It took the best part of 2 hours to cover those 15 miles even though we were all in good shape that morning. No indication of all this was mentioned in the route guide, which surprised us because, for an inexperienced bike rider, the descents in particular could prove dangerous, even in the dry. Tackling them in the wet just didn't bear thinking about. (Or were we all just getting past it?)

We bade Cornwall adieu and immersed ourselves in the rolling Devon countryside taking advantage of the brisk chuff-wind to make up for the lost time. Devon was beautiful and quite a lot of our route was familiar to me having spent a couple of holidays there. However, knowing where the most demanding hills were (like on the B3227 near South Molton) didn't, regrettably, make them any easier.

A Very Good Pud.

We stopped for lunch in Great Torrington where we found the perfect eatery at the back of the Pannier Market. We were able to leave the bikes against a wall in the old glass roofed market hall in full view of the café, which drew us in with promise of a wide range of nourishment. Three lovely girls offered us some quality tuck amongst which was an Eton Mess dessert that was a truly magnificent example of the species. This one was a mélange of ice cream, fruit salad, strawberries and the traditional crushed meringue all shoveled into a pint glass. It was absolutely delicious and only £2.75 – a bargain! If that wasn't enough, as we left the little darlings gave us a donation for the Movers & Shakers.

A Brilliant Day

We entered Somerset, our third county, on the run into Wiveliscombe, which we reached at about 6:30, more or less the same time that we had reached Tintagel the day before. Personally, I had a brilliant day on the bike. I was fully functional the whole time and I only dropped off the back on the run in because it seemed prudent to maintain a constant pace rather than get involved in one of the "burn-ups" that are an occupational hazard of riding with the Old Ports. My confidence was building no end. A couple more days like this and I might start to rediscover sensations that had seemed long gone. It was the stuff of dreams!

Wednesday 18th June

WIVELISCOMBE (SOMERSET) TO TINTERN (MON)
MILEAGE 96M
ASCENT 4800FT

Transcript from audio-log
Woken up at 5:15 by my body clock. I set it for an early rise – although not this flaming early - as there is a threat of foul weather moving in today and the plan is to get as far into the ride as possible before it engulfs us. From the window the sky is a study of grey upon grey; dark pods, almost black, heavy with water, hurry by as if on a mission, below a ceiling of solid steel. There's a significant wind; let's hope it's blowing in the right direction but I can't tell as I don't know my orientation here and it's too overcast to get a clue from the sunrise.

Having established that my internal alarm system works, albeit a little over-enthusiastically, I could usefully check out some of my other bits. I must say, two full days in the saddle have got my legs looking fitter; all the veins are standing out and my muscle tone is much improved. I haven't seen them like this for years. They're still very skinny though; you'd find more meat on a butcher's pencil! And as for my knees, they look more than ever like dented coke cans, as an old girlfriend once described them. The exorbitantly expensive saddle I treated myself to last year is definitely proving to have been a sound investment as, praise the Lord, I'm completely chafe-free in that department.

On Guards
All our good intentions of making an early start have virtually evaporated as a result of Oz's deciding to put on mudguards. While we wait for the old boy to sort himself out it starts to drizzle that fine, soft, drenching stuff that is so popular in Wales.

Our support bus is having to park temporarily on the forecourt of a car workshop preventing the proprietor opening for business whilst the riders and their bikes jostle for places on the pavement under the shop awnings, forcing women with young children and old folk in wheelchairs out into the traffic on the busy little street. Amazingly, everyone seems to be taking it all in good part. I can't help wondering how the same scene would play out in, say, Catford.

Just as eternity began to beckon, the mudguards were declared satisfactorily assembled and we were on our way. The promised torrential rain looked imminent.

Bristol Rovers
We rode out of the drizzle, the rain held off and, against all expectation, it turned into a great biking day. A howling tail wind seduced the "heavy rollers" like Jezzer, Dangerous Dave and Bashers into upping the tempo as we crossed the Somerset levels and it wasn't long before I simply did not have the pace to keep up. But I pressed on, maintaining my own cadence and preserving my strength and, in the end, the others only had to wait a few minutes for me in Cheddar. We set off all together up the Gorge and, once over the top, the speed rose again

as we headed north-northeast into our fourth county, Avon. This signaled another testing time for me but the fact that I was still with them was gratifying because, naturally, they were getting fitter too.

We stopped for lunch in the well-manicured village of Compton Dando. The pub looked a bit 'county' and I doubted they would welcome a steamy *peloton*[8] of sweaty Lycra. How mistaken I was. We were welcomed warmly and catered for handsomely: the food was excellent. Needless to say, the highlight for me was dessert - a truly scrumptious baked apple and marmalade pudding served with custard. John and I, who just happened to be sitting apart from the others, were offered complimentary drinks by the management. We accepted, naturally, but we never discovered what we had done to deserve this extra attention.

Towards the end of the afternoon we had to find our way around Bristol but the route plan that we were following wasn't up to the task. In order to get to where we needed to be, namely on the cycle path over the Severn Road Bridge, a bit of imaginative improvisation was required. Things turned a little fractious as we struggled to navigate our way around numerous housing estates but good humours were soon restored once we picked up the scent. Crossing the Severn Bridge was quite an experience. The bridge must be hell for agoraphobics because it is very open, exposed and prone to high, gusting crosswinds. You dare not loosen your grip on the handlebars for a second.

---

[8] A bunch of cyclists

Not long after reaching the other side we descended at great speed into Tintern and the Wye Valley Hotel. We were also now in our 6th county, Monmouthshire, having clipped Gwent as we came off the Severn Bridge. By the time we arrived at 5:30 our cycle-computers showed that we'd covered 96 miles yet I was still so full of riding. The dream continued. Our luck with hotel grub held for another night so, all in all it turned out to be pretty good day.

Thursday 19th June

TINTERN (MONS) TO MUCH WENLOCK (SHROPSHIRE)
MILEAGE 83M
ASCENT 5300FT

The stormy rain forecast for the previous day didn't arrive until after we got to the hotel: perfect timing! It then blew itself out over night leaving us with a bright, sunny day for our ride through the Welsh border country to Much Wenlock. The breakfast menu was rather limited and I made the mistake again of allowing myself to be tempted by bacon and eggs. I very soon regretted it. Within 10 minutes of leaving Tintern we encountered a 1 in 7 (14%) climb, which went on for what seemed like miles and highlighted the fact that my left leg wasn't functioning properly again.

Fortunately that proved to be the only serious climb of the day and the rest of the ride was more in keeping with the terrain that our training circuits in Kent and Surrey offer, i.e. plenty of hills but nothing that forced us to chew our handlebars. (This is not to suggest that the southeast doesn't have its share of stiff ones; we just didn't go looking for them as a rule.) This widening of the contours enabled me to hang on until lunchtime when my body had an opportunity to switch itself on fully.

The Lady and the Sharp Dressed Man
During lunch Peter and I got talking to an unusual couple, who expressed considerable interest in our cause.

They had turned up in a collector's item - a 1970s Jaguar XJ-S Estate - only, the state of this particular example suggested that the pair might not be the world's most fanatical classic car enthusiasts. The vehicle appeared to have been jet-washed with the contents of a muck spreader and the interior showed all the signs that it accommodated assorted livestock on a regular basis. The woman wore a stylish mackintosh buttoned to the chin: curious, given that the day was, by then, sunny and warm. She seemed a little jaded and frayed around the edges, yet her fine complexion and the twinkle in her eyes suggested that she once enjoyed more glamorous, uplifting times.

Her companion, in contrast, closely resembled one of the front men in ZZ Top and was dressed as a cowboy from the Stetson on his head to the Cuban heeled riding boots on his feet. We gave them a set of leaflets, which the woman insisted she would follow up when she got home. When we had to go I said goodbye with considerable regret. They clearly had a story to tell, which I would have dearly loved to hear.

Our first mishap of the ride occurred just outside Ludlow when John Mulvaney crashed on a gravelly corner. He donated a fair amount of skin to the District Council and it all looked very painful. But once we'd straightened up his bike he was able to ride gently into the town where we commandeered a seat in the market square to administer first aid to his open wounds and apply ice lollies to his bruises. (Don't bother looking for this procedure in the paramedic code of practice).

An Evening in Heaven

That afternoon was a revelation for me. I felt terrific and experienced the sort of physical freedom that had been missing for so long. I couldn't remember feeling better on a bike in 30 years. I was ecstatic as we flew into a Much Wenlock that was bathed in golden, late afternoon sunshine. A day to savour but there was more delight yet to come in the shape of our accommodation for the night. The Fox Inn was superbly comfortable and reputed to be the best restaurant in town. And I'm sure it was. If the starters and main dishes were top quality then the hands of angels made the desserts. The bread and butter pudding was simply the best that I've ever tasted. My only gripe was that it wasn't twice the size.

Prior to the meal, two of my very old friends, Tim and Annabel, and their two boys, paid us a visit. They popped down from Shrewsbury where Tim is Head of Geography at Shrewsbury School. They stayed with us for aperitifs but were unable to remain for the evening. That was a shame because both Tim and Annie possessed impressive sporting credentials, which would have surely led to some interesting exchanges had they been able to dine with us. Tim had been an international high jumper and was UK champion and record holder in the early 1980s and

Annie had competed successfully as a rower and made a mark in Concept 2 indoor competition.

It would have been particularly apt to spend the evening in Much Wenlock discussing athletics and athleticism given the little town's very special association with sport. It was hard to believe that the multi-billion dollar, global bun fight that would be opening in Beijing in a little over a month owed its existence to the vision and action of a son of Much Wenlock, Dr. William Penny Brookes. He introduced physical education into British schools and in the mid 1800s organized his "Olympian" games in the town in order to "promote moral, physical and intellectual improvement" amongst the town's inhabitants.

These games became internationally renowned and attracted the attention of Frenchman Baron Pierre de Coubertain who was so inspired by what he saw he went away and revived the classical games of ancient Greece and staged his version 6 years later in 1896 in Athens. The rest, as they say, is (also) history.

The local games are alive and well and continue to be held in the town every July: definitely one for the diary.

Friday 20th June

MUCH WENLOCK (SHROPSHIRE)
TO ALTRINCHAM (GREATER MANCHESTER)
MILEAGE 76.5M
ASCENT 2280FT

Frilly Knickers

We set off towards Altrincham at about 9 o'clock following a bit of banter with the governor at the hotel who suggested that we'd left something behind in one of the rooms. He then produced a pair of frilly knickers and handcuffs: a real character and a superb venue.

It was overcast as we pulled out of Much Wenlock and headed for the Wrekin, a particularly vicious lump, at least from a cyclist's point of view, on the Shropshire landscape. Thankfully, however, traveling in the direction we were going meant we descended its formidable side.

A former Celtic fort and capital of the Cornovii people, this bronze age site has remained one of the few places in England that retains a name of Celtic origin. At 1300 feet it dominates the surrounding countryside for miles and can be seen from as far away as Manchester in the north and Gloucester to the south.

As its height suggested, the descent of the Wrekin down to the Shropshire Plain was long, almost alpine like, with many bends made all the more tricky for us by the arrival of the long-promised rain.

Call it what you will – nerve, bravura, skill or simply madness, but cyclists have it in varying degrees when it comes to descending hills. Our little group is no exception. At one end of the scale is big Jezzer who seems prepared to launch himself headlong down any gradient, rain or shine, while at the other is yours truly who struggles to prevent an ectomorphic body and gossamer bike from becoming airborne when impacting uneven road surfaces. Not surprisingly, therefore, we all arrive at the base of the ancient mound separately each coming down the mighty hill in his own sweet way.

Dicing With Death

Once reassembled, we set off in a northerly direction towards Market Drayton with all thoughts of woad now limited to the tarmac one ahead. The south westerlies were still backing us so progress was swift and we were once again blessed by a change in the weather. Away scudded the rain clouds and another bright sunny day was ours in which to enjoy a series of gently rolling roads dotted with pretty villages through lush, arable farmland. We were able to maintain a brisk tempo virtually all day, until, that is, we crossed into Greater Manchester. This coincided with the beginning of the rush hour and we found ourselves having to switch riding mode from *Audax* (long distance cycle-touring) to *criterium racing* (frenetic, short circuit with constant sprints) in order to cope in the precarious and unpredictable world of cyclo-commuting.

Our arrival in Manchester was doubly fraught because our route instructions again proved to be of little help in finding our hotel. It's one thing mixing it with commuter traffic, indeed it can be fun, but it's another thing doing it when you don't know where you are going. Having to make split-second changes in direction midway through negotiating multi-laned junctions and roundabouts is not conducive to maintaining rude health nor to keeping the seat of your shorts fresh.

Crash Test Dummy

It was at this stage that John crashed again. He had glanced at his map just as we were passing through a width-restricting traffic-calming measure and had run straight into the curb having failed to notice the changing line of the pavement. You had to hand it to the local highway engineers; their system worked very well. It sure slowed us down. This time John's injuries really did look nasty. He had taken the brunt of the fall on the same elbow as the day before and there was real fear that it might now be broken. The cloud surrounding John's misfortune did, however, have one sizable patch of silver lining: it gave Jezzer and Bashers an opportunity to waylay a couple of passing schoolboys to help locate our hotel. They obviously did a fine job between them because we seemed to ride straight there once we'd got John moving again.

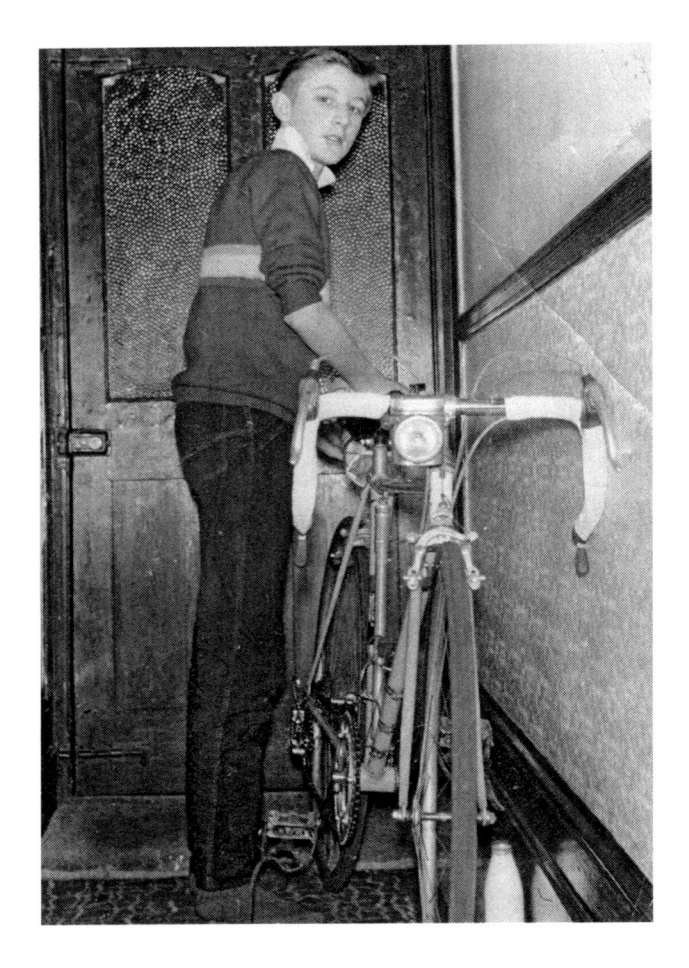

*At 14 with my first racing bike
- and Billy Fury haircut to verify the year - 1958.*

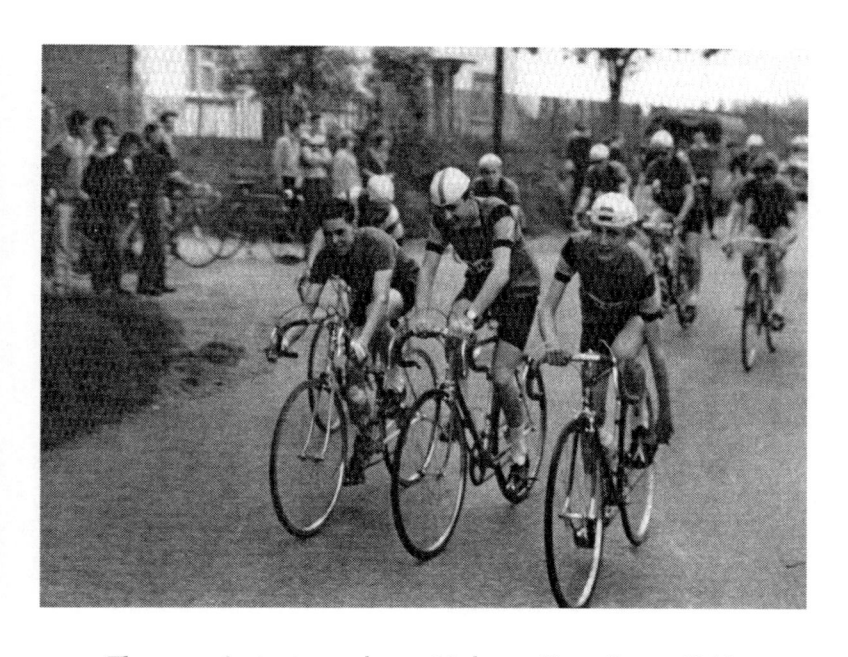

*The start of a junior road race. Higham, Kent. Spring 1962.
Posn. DNF (collided with a horse!)*

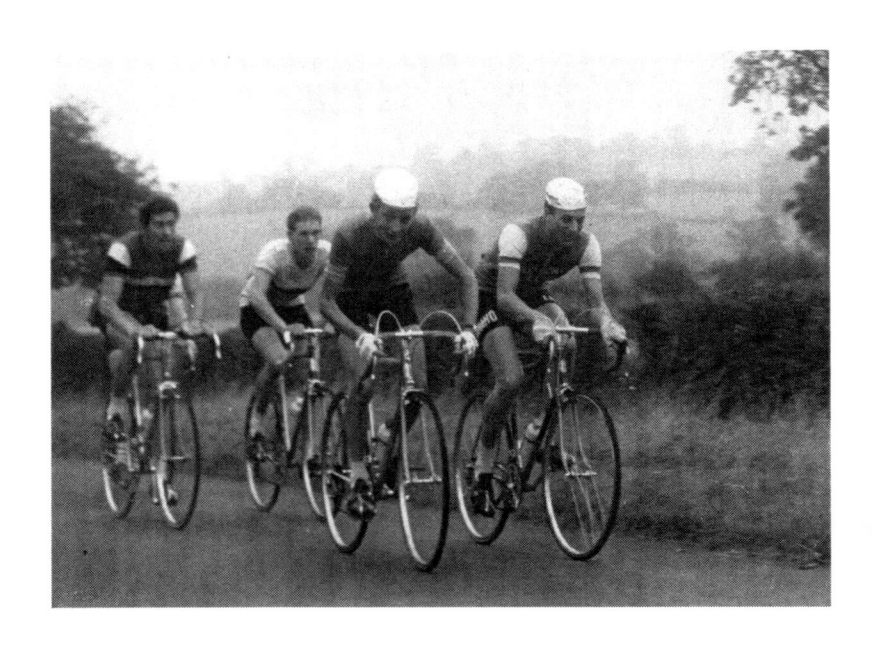

Setting the pace in Essex. October 1963. Posn. 6th

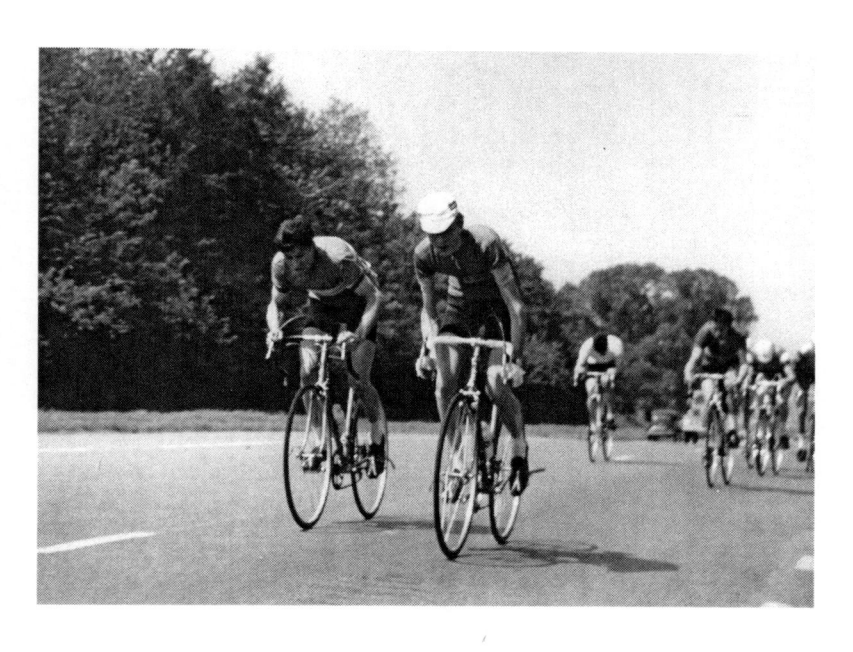

Sprinting for the line. Higham.
Summer 1964 Posn. 3rd

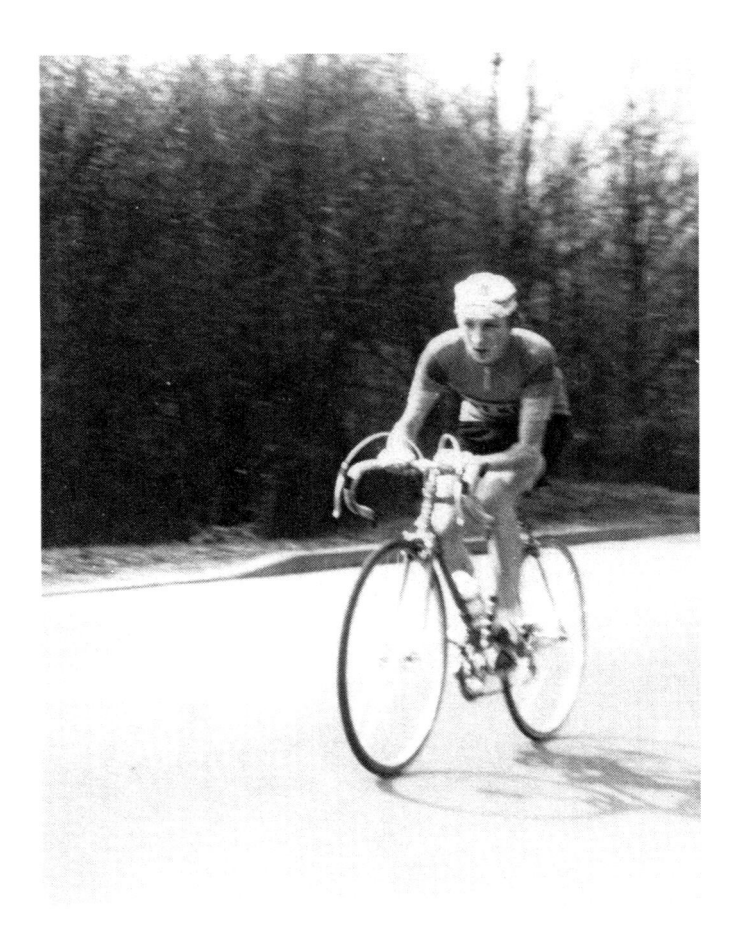

Lone breakaway to victory. Longfield, Kent September 1963

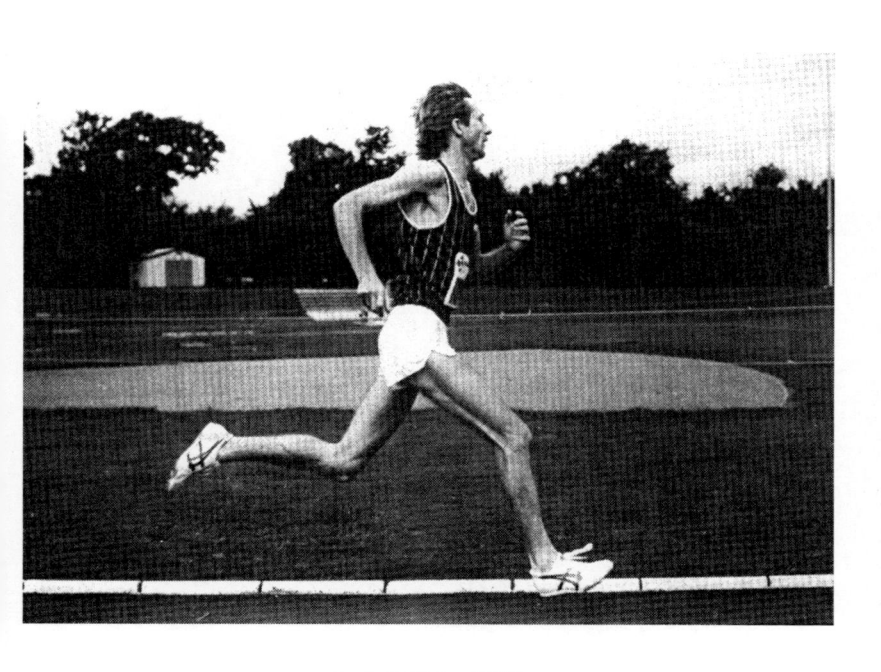

In full flight 1986

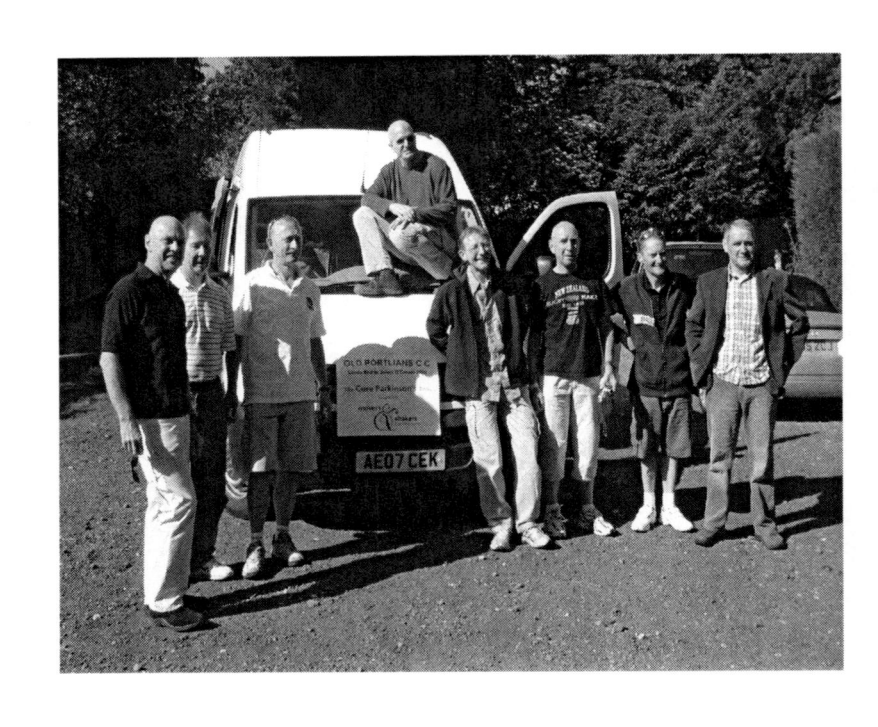

The unlikely lads about to leave Hayes

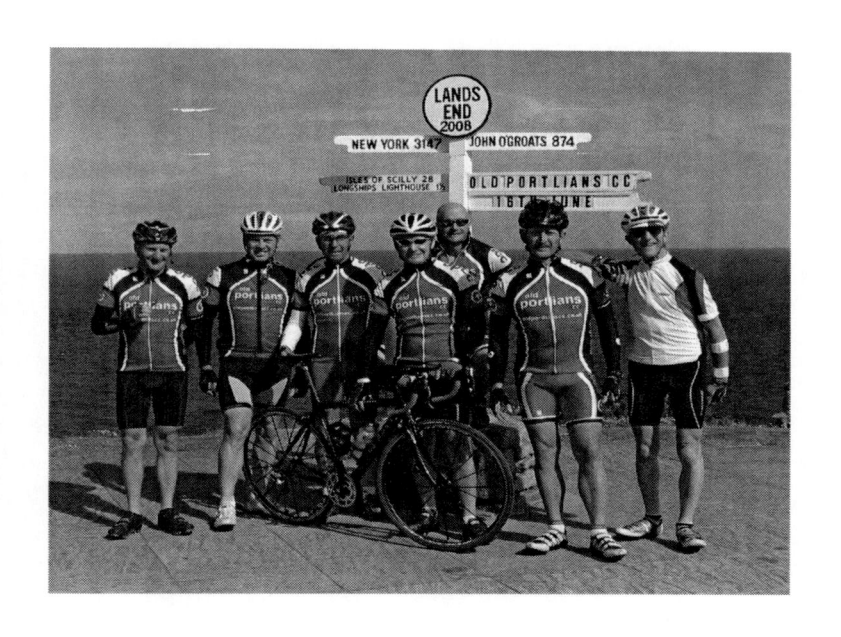

Left to right - Oz, Dave, Barry, John, Jezzer, Bashers and the author.

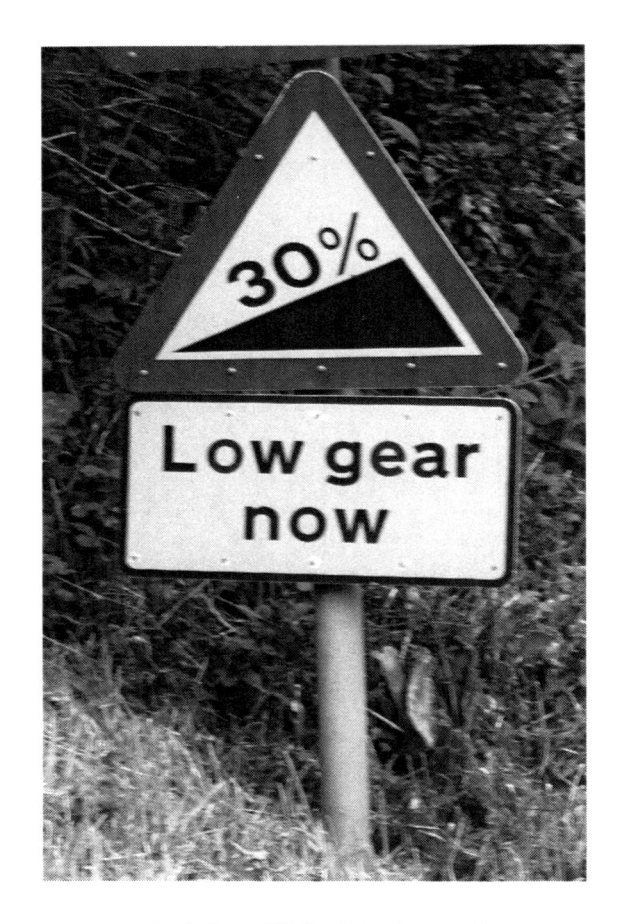

the "Great Wall of Crackington"

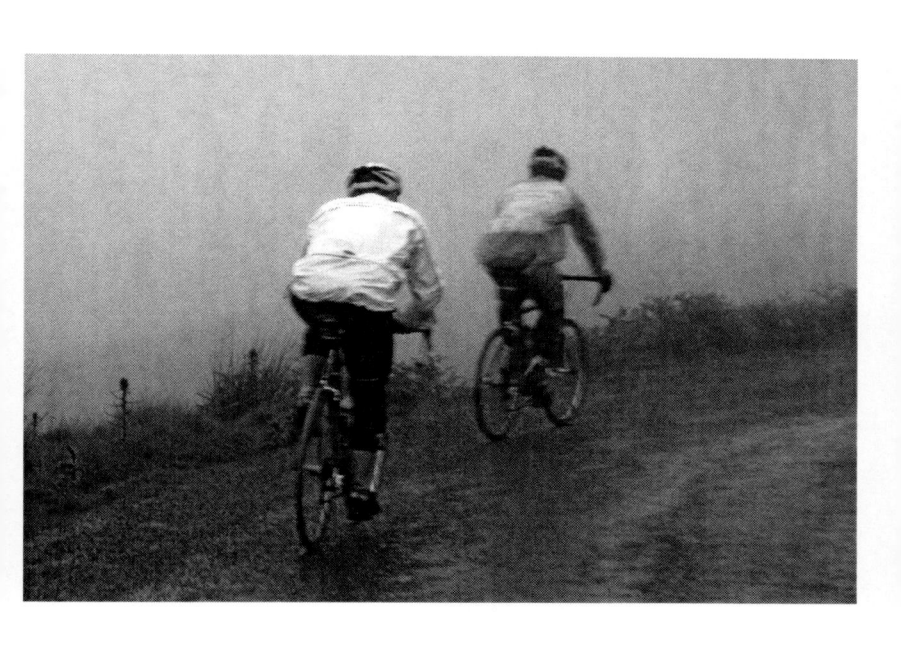

... and this is the scenic route!

*Recuperating at the Temple Sowerby Rescue Centre
aka The Kings Arms Hotel*

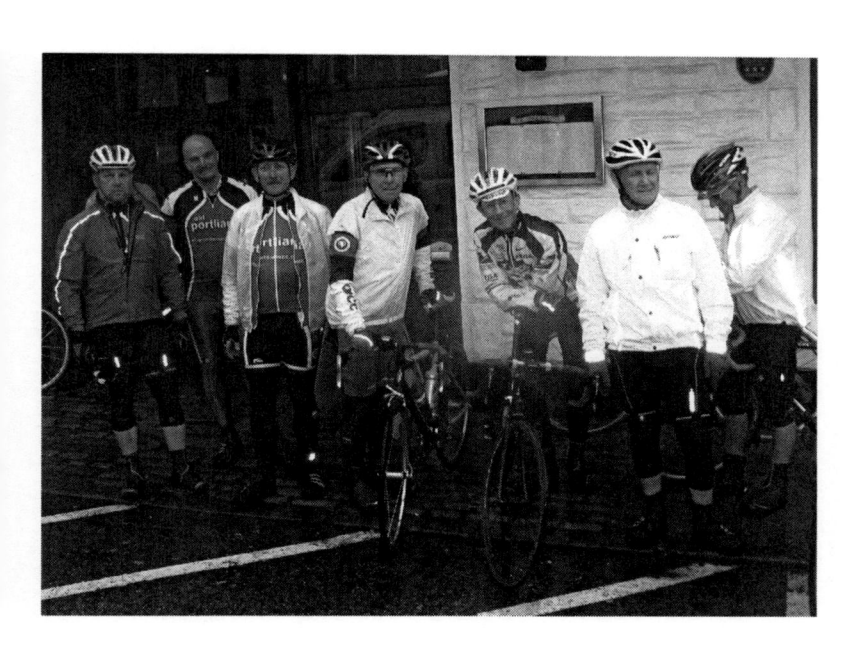

Cairngorms here we come

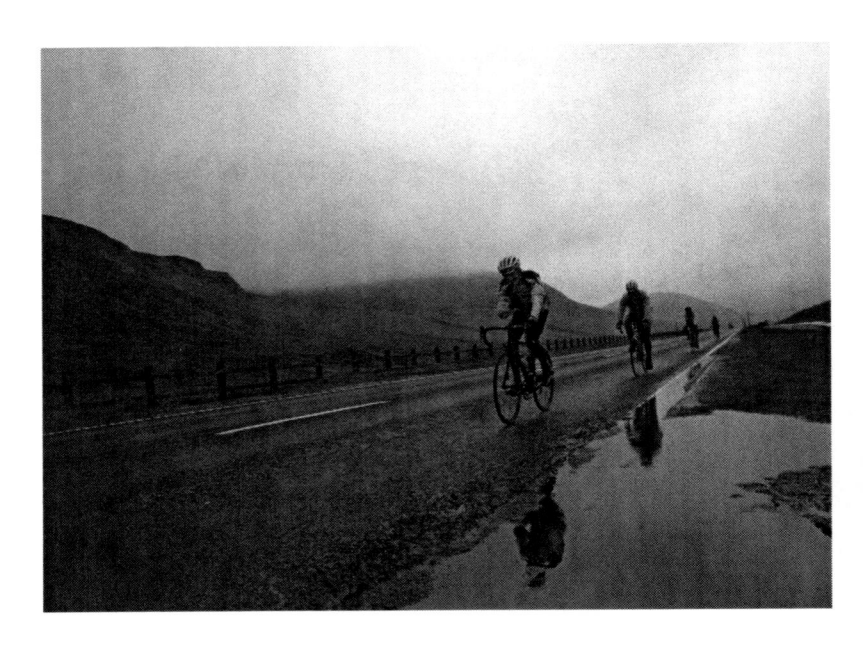

Oh, the joy of cycling.

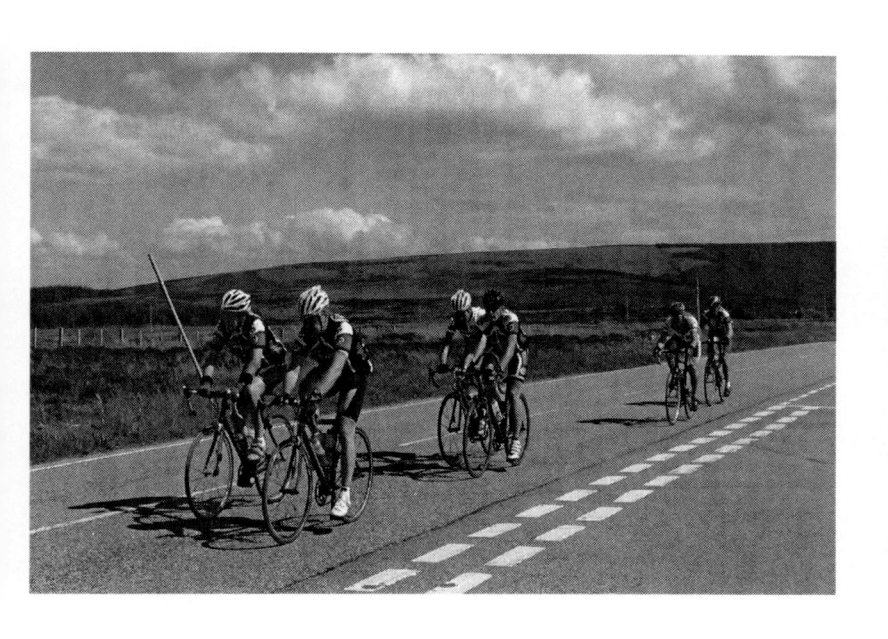

En route to Crask Inn. It doesn't get much better than this.

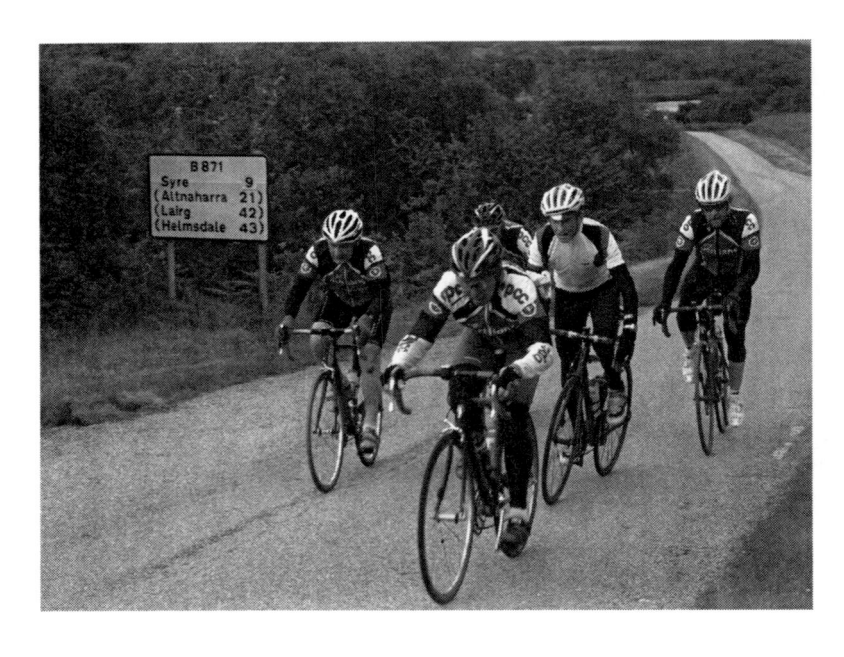

Getting the power down through Strath Naver.

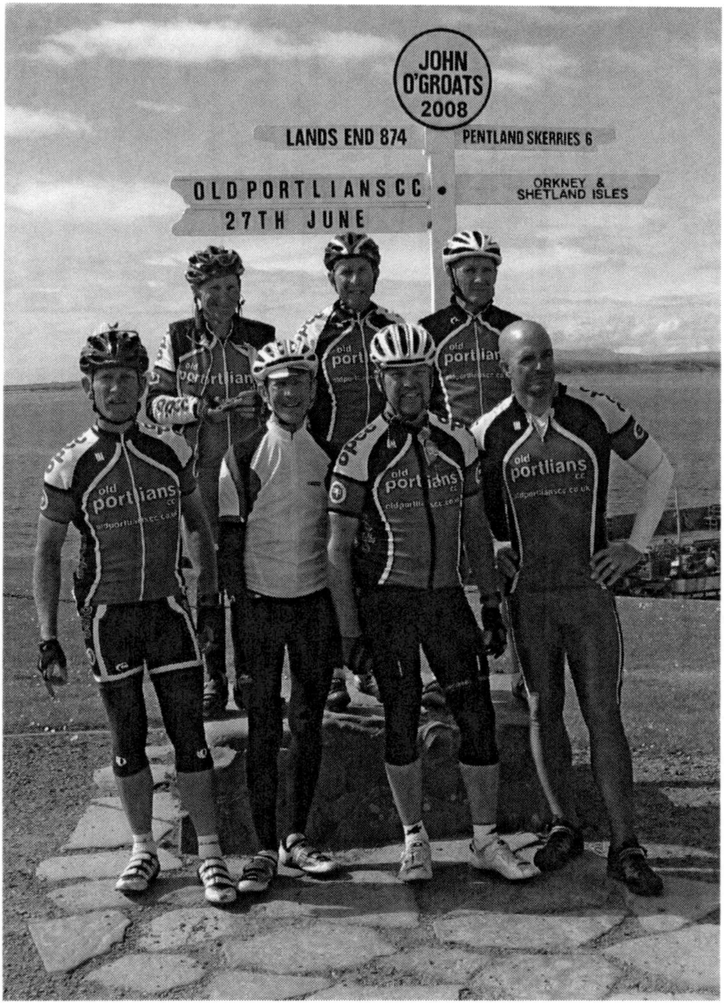
JOHN
O'GROATS
2008
LANDS END 874
PENTLAND SKERRIES 6
OLDPORTLIANSCC
27TH JUNE
ORKNEY &
SHETLAND ISLES

On arrival, the first job was to get John examined by a first-aider who took one look at his arm and insisted that he be taken to the local small injuries clinic. He got back just before dinner, heavily bandaged, brandishing a ten-pound note and with the good news that nothing was broken. He would be with us on our push into North Yorkshire on the morrow. And the tenner? – a donation to the CPT from the clinic.

Saturday 21st June

Altrincham (Greater Manchester) to High Bentham (North Yorkshire)
Mileage 80m
Ascent 6520ft

40 Miles of Bad Road

This section of the route would take us up onto the North Yorkshire Moors via the Trough of Bowland and Slaidburn and was potentially going to be the toughest day so far. It was only to be expected, therefore, that this should be the day that the rain finally caught up with us. It poured and, as had been forecast, it was cold and windy which meant we had to clad ourselves in full winter gear. The first couple of hours were spent negotiating our way northwards through the suburbs of Greater Manchester where the road surfaces were in appalling condition. I have no recollection of where we stopped for lunch but it would have been somewhere north of Blackburn between Mellor and Whalley. We did, of course, appreciate the opportunity to get in out of the downpour for a while but putting cold, clammy togs on again and stepping back into the deluge was the unpleasant price we had to pay for that all too brief spell of relative comfort. The rain continued to bucket down whilst the terrain grew more hostile.

Just north of Clitheroe on the B6478 we climbed up the side of Eagle Fell (maximum gradient 1 in 6 or 17%) before descending equally steeply into Newton in Bowland in the Hodder Valley. Then it was up another

1 in 6 into Slaidburn where we turned onto a narrow mountain road that climbed for the best part of 5 miles over Catlow Fell (1600 feet) before dropping down to High Bentham.

Look, No Hands

We had been out for over 8 hours under what felt like a cold power shower and for the final couple of hours we had the added delight of being shrouded in swirling mist. It was, without doubt, one of the grimmest day's cycling that I have ever experienced. My hands went completely numb so that changing gear and braking became something of a lottery. Another hazard was the frequent occurrence of cattle grids although I couldn't be worrying about those; the weather and terrain were enough to cope with already. Apart from making sure that I approached them at 90 degrees, I just hit the metal slats at full tilt. This seemed to work; I just had to hope my wheels were up to it.

Some years ago I cycled 50 miles alone through the tail end of a typhoon in the hills of the Coramandel Peninsular in New Zealand. It was an awesome experience riding in the heaviest rain I have ever witnessed that turned long stretches of what was already a difficult highway into an almost impassable sea of clay. The lightening was incredible; it seemed to ground within yards of me and was followed immediately by claps of thunder that reverberated right through to my soul. But despite the solitude, the potential danger and the Danté-esque conditions of that ride I don't remember feeling as uncomfortable and miserable as I did at times on the road to High Bentham.

The Nobel Prize for Humanity

We eventually reached our destination at about 6 o'clock. It wasn't obvious where the digs were, so whilst we fathomed that out, we all fell into what was, unquestionably, the most welcomed sight of the day: The Coach House Inn. The proprietor was one of the many lovely people that we met on the trip who I would recommend for the Nobel Prize for Humanity. She made us most welcome and plied us with hot tea and coffee until we had thawed out. But the nightmare wasn't quite over. Our beds for the night were still another couple of damp, hilly miles down the road to which we contrived to add another mile with a detour down a lane that turned into a boulder-strewn track to nowhere. The day seemed determined to break our spirit and, as we bumped and slithered our way back up the track with still no firm idea of where we were in relation to our accommodation, it got close to succeeding. Fortunately, on getting back to the road, we found New Butts Farm languishing in the gloom less than 50m beyond the junction. If only we had overshot that lane like we had so many others in the last few days.

The B&B was adequate but didn't offer much in the way of facilities. Most unfortunate was the scarcity of showers and toilets. We really could have done with more sumptuous surroundings after a day like that. Still, we had a good meal back in the Coach House where my friends Fiona and Paul and Fiona's two boys, Tom and Frank, my godsons, joined us. They had traveled over from Leeds for the weekend specifically to meet us. The boys, aged 11 and 8, got on really well with the gang - but I suppose that wasn't surprising given that we were all children at heart. Everyone enjoyed an excellent evening, which did much to restore morale. Once I'd had time to reflect I realised that, despite everything, I had fared pretty well again and had been able to keep the pedals turning purposefully right through to the end. I just hoped I could do the same again the next day, which was going to be a long one.

Sunday 22nd June

High Bentham (North Yorkshire) to Langholm (Dumfries & Galloway)
Mileage 102m   Ascent 6900ft

The weather forecast for the 100 plus miles through North Yorkshire, Cumbria and across the border into Dumfries and Galloway was for a continuation of gales and periods of torrential rain. In view of this, I took the precaution of calling a close friend who had lived for many years near Kirby Lonsdale to get his reaction to our proposed route. He confirmed that we would have to return to the high moorlands again via Kingsdale and Deepdale before dropping down into Dentdale, Sedburgh and on to the Lune Valley.

I had spent quite a bit of time in this part of the world and so I knew how lovely this road could be when the sun shone but as it was, it would mean more of what we had had to endure the previous day. So we decided to head straight to Kirby Lonsdale into the strong, gusting wind and turn north there on the A683 to Sedburgh, which gave us the benefit of a tailwind again boosting our progress through the Lune Valley and beyond.

I had been looking forward to bowling through the cultivated farmlands of the valley with the mountains in the distance on either side: to the left - the Lakeland

Fells and to the right - the Pennines. But in the present conditions that, too, offered little.

Had the weather not been so extreme I would have suggested taking a short detour for a morning coffee in the Tebay Service Area on the M6 (it is not always appreciated that service areas have non-motorway tradesmen's entrances) so that my companions could experience the phenomenon of a motorway service area in the UK serving well prepared, healthy food at sensible prices in a pleasant and relaxing setting where people actually chose to go to dine out. Can you imagine taking your loved-one to Watford Gap or Hilton Park for a slap-up? You'd be guaranteed a slap down, that's for sure.

Hitching A Ride

The wind grew stronger and the rain turned spiteful, stinging our faces. Then, as we rode through Tebay itself, I was side-swiped by an almighty gust that blew me into the gutter and onto the grass verge: the spot I would have chosen given the alternatives of curb or puddled carriageway. In the next town, Orton, we took a B road that paralleled the M6 as it climbed over Shap Summit. Normally, this would have been one of the notable climbs of the whole E2E trip but such was the strength of the tailwind we were able to make light of it. However, near the top, as we stopped to regroup, my bike was once again blown away from beneath me and, for a moment, I could see it heading for Scotland on its own. Fortunately I managed to stymie this heroic bid for freedom by just catching hold of the rear wheel.

The wind was gale force now and, although it was going our way, the gusts were unpredictable and its sheer power unnerving. We continued over the murky top to where Peter and Steve had parked up. The countryside here is completely exposed and away from the lee of the bus it was a real struggle to stay afoot. Opening and closing the bus doors also offered something of a challenge. We later learnt that the Met Office had issued special warnings for the region that day and the M6 motorway had been closed at Shap because of the severe conditions!

The group decided that, in the interest of my health and safety and their peace of mind, I should travel down the mountain in the bus. The descent was unknown territory and there was genuine concern about my lack of ballast in such extreme conditions (man and bike combined – a strapping 65 kilos!). As if there wasn't enough for us all to contend with, we then realized that Jezzer, who had ridden off ahead of the rest of us, was unlikely to have spotted the turning we now needed to take and was probably at that moment plummeting at great speed down into Appleby, a nice town but not at all where we wanted to be on this occasion. So, whilst Dangerous, Bashers, Father Jack, Disco and Oz took the allotted route down the hillside, the bus, with me on board chased after Jezzer, eventually finding him sheltering in the bushes on the outskirts of

Appleby. We then retraced to the summit and followed the way taken by the others.

The bus made its way down to Temple Sowerby where Peter brokered a deal with the landlady of the King's Arms Hotel for the use of the pub's facilities, particularly her tumble dryer. The lady was a saint! Nothing was too much trouble. She even set aside a games room for our exclusive use as a changing room. (She would also be going on my list of Nobel Prize nominees.) Dry and warm, we assemble in the bar for some hot food. It had seemed a long morning but we had yet to reach halfway for the day.

Scheduled as 90-odd miles, this stage was going to exceed 100. The wind was still very strong, but with our being at a much lower elevation now meant that it was far more predictable and manageable; certainly enough for me to resume riding. Apart from when the wind decided to pick on me, I had been riding well in the morning and my form continued into the afternoon. Towards the end of the day, however, weariness did start to get the better of me and it was a case of shutting out everything I didn't need and focusing on getting by. It was at times like this that the lads really came into their own - reassuring, cajoling, waiting, encouraging and generally pulling me through. On the face of it, we were an incongruous lot but, on this trip, cometh the hour, we operated as harmoniously as anyone could wish.

Bike Bits

When we eventually reached our destination we discovered that our lodgings offered the added bonus of a well-equipped workshop, which the landlord was happy for us to use. This was a real stroke of luck as it meant that we would be able to pay some long-overdue attention to our bikes, working in relative comfort. Jezzer had broken his chain the day before, twice in fact, and had eventually been persuaded that nothing short of a new set of sprockets and chain would do. He needed a surprising amount of convincing though. After all, the present block and chain had only done Paris-Brest-Paris and all the training leading up to it!

Given that amount of mileage and considering the giga-Newtons that this man Jezzer was capable of forcing through his drive-train, it was a miracle that his top tube hadn't bifurcated his progenitoria long before. Both Disco and I had completely worn out a set of brake blocks each over the previous two days and it was highly improbable that Dangerous's bike was without need of some new part or adjustment. Peter and Steve had made a detour via Kendal first thing that morning to pick up all the bits that everyone needed. The workshop looked set to become a hive of industry.

By the time we'd shaken ourselves down, spruced ourselves up and were ready to down a few glasses of the local '70

Shilling' ale at a nearby hotel, it had begun to pour down again. The elements just had to have the last say!

*"I specifically said 'pour down' there because if you've had any association at all with north of the border you will be familiar with the constant references to how often it "pours **up**" in Scotland. Given the number of deluges that I've encountered north of the border over the years you would have thought, simply by the law of averages, that I would have experienced at least a little of this amazing phenomenon of precipitation heading skywards, but, alas, I haven't. Earthbound rods of water do, from time to time, bounce up off the tarmac a couple of centimeters when the elements go into monsoon mode and it could be argued that, for those briefest of moments, the rain was defying gravity. But I'll be very disappointed if that's all there is to it.*

Advice on a postcard, please...

How I Miss Nostalgia.

The bar in the hotel was pokey and showed signs of stress to the point of distress; the same went for the local clientele (except "pokey", of course. I don't think I've ever come across a "pokey" person; I wouldn't know what to look for, really.) The place had undoubtedly been witness to countless acts of cognitive obfuscation and self-annihilation over the years and the whole bar scene reminded me of the venues that I used to frequent during the "pub-rock" era in London in the late 60s/early 70s to "take in" bands like Dr. Feelgood, Brinsley Schwarz, Mickey Jupp, Ducks Deluxe ... ah, halcyon days.

A couple of pints later, our confidence in the hotel being able to provide us with food beyond a few bags of deep-fried haggis scratchings, had waned. However, it was pointed out to us that there was a restaurant downstairs and that they were expecting us. Our host at the B&B had very thoughtfully and prudently alerted the pub to an impending assault on their kitchen by nine famished Sassenachs. Good man.

Happy Ever 'Afters'
Downstairs is a different world and both the main menu and the dessert board show signs of invention and creativity. The list of puds will require particularly lengthy deliberation when the time comes. My dilemma will be whether to go for a traditional old favorite, like syrup sponge, custard and/ or ice cream (preferably 'and') or try something new and gamble on it being sufficiently clarty and bulky to satisfy the appetite of a growing lad on a bike. Decision time: I feel like flirting with recklessness tonight and plump for novelty - the apricot and dark chocolate meringue. Although this pudding is based on a confection of near zero substance and that there is, therefore, high probability of my leaving the table less than satiated, just the thought of the marriage of those flavours and textures has sent my taste buds into orbit and rendered the dish irresistible. All fears that it might prove inadequate are, however, dispelled as it is served. It is

the size of a grapefruit and full of dark chocolate ice cream – choc-full, you might say. Great call!

It had been a long, eventful day with something for the masochist and the aesthete alike. During the storm, before our body and soul-saving lunchtime sojourn in the Temple Sowerby Health Spa (a-k-a the King's Arms Hotel), we had passed through the halfway point of our *Grande Epreuve* in terms of mileage. With 7 days down and just 5 to go, this suggested that we still had some long days ahead of us.

Monday 23rd June

Langholm (Dumfries & Galloway) to Dunfirmline (Fife) Mileage 90m Ascent 4720ft

Bashers installed himself down in the workshop long before anyone else had stirred and had got on with fixing the various problems with the bikes. It was very good of him to take on so much of the work but I suspect there was a sizeable chunk of self-interest in his generosity – he probably didn't have much faith in the technical competence of the rest of us and could see the jobs dragging on into the morning or worse, finding himself having to get his tools out on a bleak mountainside somewhere. As we fuelled up at the breakfast table the weather report came on the radio confirming that, contrary to previous predictions, we would enjoy a dry, bright day before the return of the wet and windy conditions for the rest of the week; the news sparked little reaction. We had assumed at the beginning of the trip that the weather forecast would be essential listening but more often than not the forecasts had proven unreliable. We had been promised foul, stormy conditions ever since leaving Cornwall but they didn't materialize until we left Manchester on day 6. So, having braced ourselves in readiness for a continuation of the weekend's desperate weather, there we were facing the prospect of another lovely sunny day. How unsettling is that?

Except for the first day out of Land's End, one thing that had remained more or less constant was the wind direction. This morning it whisked us over the luxuriant and rolling countryside of Eskdale at a very respectable pace so that by lunchtime we had covered the 50+ miles to Peebles, a truly delightful town that immediately struck me as somewhere I would like to visit again when I was free of time constraints, lycra and "clackety" shoes.

Up until the 1960s, Peebles was very much part of the Border Country's wool industry but since then it has become home to a growing number of people who travel into Edinburgh to work. The town's popularity with commuters is easy to understand. In just the time it has taken us to ride into the centre of the town, locate a suitable hostelry, have lunch and proceed out the other side, I have picked up a distinct, pervasive air of bonhomie and well-being, which is borne out by my subsequent discovery that a British, independent think-tank, 'The New Economics Foundation', within the last four years, voted Peebles top town in Scotland (2nd in the UK) for its range of independent traders and its ability to preserve a "home-town identity". I want to go back there even more now. Hebdon Bridge was the UK #1, in case you are wondering.

For my money, this was the most scenic day of the trip so far. In parts, the verdant undulations reminded me of the North and South Downs but on a larger scale. The pleasure afforded by the surrounding countryside coupled with the exhilaration of riding fluidly and easily made this a special day. As we approached Edinburgh we became increasingly caught up in the hurly burly of the big city at a busy time of the day, much as we had done on the runs into Manchester and Bristol. Happily, though, this time our trail, admirably blazed by captain Bashers, took us along wide, well-signed roads. It was only when we caught sight of the Firth of Forth that complications set in. For the casual, non-motorized user, motorway bridges invariably prove substantial stumbling blocks to progress. Indeed, you could be forgiven for thinking that there was a move to actively discourage pedestrians and cyclists from using them so fiendishly tortuous are the networks of cycle and walkways that serve them. Had it not been such a bright, sunny evening, frustration might have got the better of us but, in the event, we managed to find our way on to the bridge soon enough for our collective composure to remain intact.

As we emerged from the trees on the bank onto the beginning of the open span, the view was truly magnificent. To our left, looking westwards stretched the upper reaches of the Firth. To the north, straight ahead, lay Fife with what I guessed were the Ochills, and/or the Sidlaw Hills forming the horizon. But, most spectacular of all, immediately to our right, loomed the original Forth Bridge in all its red oxide glory.

By the time we reached our digs in Dunfirmline, we had clocked up 90 miles for the day. I was still enjoying good form and had even experienced flashbacks to what I had felt like in former times. My PD was barely an issue. That evening we ate in a local bar/bistro/diner where, almost to a man, we chose the spaghetti and meatballs; just what the doctor ordered to restock the old mitochondria after a long day on the bike depleting them. Then it was a couple of quick drinks before retiring early to bed. We were definitely in "midge country" now so it was time to get out the much-vaunted *Avon Skin-so-Soft* moisturising spray. Hitherto I hadn't had an opportunity to try it as an insect repellant but I had used it successfully to remove oil from a pair of white socks the previous day.

*For a comprehensive list of the alternative
uses of this product log onto
www.kitchencraftsnmore.net/skinsosoft.html*

Tuesday 24ᵗ June

Dunfirmline (Fife) to Blairgowrie (Perthshire)
Mileage 60m
Ascent 3080ft

A relatively short, straightforward day lay ahead - at least that was the theory. According to our host, rain was due and would linger in the north-east keeping it chilly while the rest of the British Isles continued to enjoy wall-to-wall sunshine with temperatures in the high 70s.

Wrong time, wrong place, again! You can bet your life that if my ship ever comes in, I shall be waiting at the airport.

The Key To It All
Just as we had done on a couple of previous occasions when poor weather had threatened, we tried to make an early start in order to get as far down the road as possible before the elements caught up with us. But, just as before, we failed, hopelessly. When the moment came to return our room keys I couldn't find mine. We searched high and low through all the rooms, bags and the bus and even revisited the bistro where we'd been the previous evening but to no avail. The problem was that the keys also gave access to the house so if they didn't turn up all the locks in the whole place would have to be changed. It was such a relief therefore when the keys were found among some items of washing that the lady of the house had done for me earlier that morning. Phew!

Give and Take

While everyone else was hunting for the key, Bashers used the time wisely, to "re-evaluate" the official itinerary, removing a couple of what we all subsequently agreed were pointless loops. Unfortunately we then contrived to get lost and ended up adding miles back on so that the day's tally of just over 60 miles was more or less the same distance as originally scheduled. Nevertheless, compared to all the other days, leaving aside a long 1 in 5 hill, which caused a certain amount of grief about an hour into the day's ride, this was a saunter. It was just a pity that Bashers hadn't spotted that hill first thing and found a way to "re evaluate" that, too.

Our journey northwards into Tayside saw us passing through places with great names that sounded like characters from a Mervyn Peake story – Yetts O'Muckhart, Findo Gask, Fowlis Wester and Moneydie. I couldn't help wondering how these names originated and what tosses the cabers of these places nowadays, so to speak. I also tried to envisage the type of character Peake might have created for each one but decided to save that for a rainy day. I didn't have to wait long for one of those but with the rain came much else to occupy my mind so the exercise was never undertaken. Another time, perhaps…

We reached Blairgowrie by early afternoon. It had been a mostly overcast day but the rain, once again, defied the experts and stayed aloft.

Wednesday 25th June

Blairgowrie (Perthshire) to Nairn (Highlands)
Mileage 102m
Ascent 7200ft

Transcript from audiolog
Setback.
I've had something of a setback. I've tweaked my lower back. It happens from time to time, usually if I pick up something awkwardly, which is what I did yesterday morning whilst searching for that confounded key! It's something to do with having a hyper-mobile facet joint at L4 or L5. Anyway, suffice it to say the pain is severely restricting my ability to get around and in particular to negotiate the transitions between sitting and standing. Oddly, but mercifully, the dodgy back doesn't seem to affect me once I'm on the bike. At least, that was the case yesterday but it was very painful dismounting and moving about afterwards and it is very sparky again this morning. I therefore got up early to give myself time to stretch it out; it seems to help. I suppose I'll have to add these exercises to the other tiresome rituals that I have to perform each morning before entering the public domain, like counting and dividing the day's pills and potions, and distributing them around my many pockets so that they are accessible every hour and a half whilst I am in the saddle. It's been one thing after another. I'm beginning to think I am not meant to succeed in this mission. My resolve is being tested to the hilt for some reason. I expect a nudge from the Parkinson's if I get too cocky about things, but on this trip so far its interventions have been scarce and largely incidental. All the difficulties and discomfort that I have been getting

are from relatively new issues I hadn't originally bargained for. "The irony of fate", I suppose.

The rain was teeming down as we rolled away from the hotel and headed northwards once again towards the Cairngorms.

This was the day we had all feared but, taking the day as a whole, it perhaps wasn't so bad and we managed, in the end, to cover the 100+ miles in a fairly respectable time. Along the way, however, there were some dire periods when the long, seemingly endless and often brutal climbs took us up above the cloud base and along roads that had even the redoubtable Jezzer groaning and cursing. The effort that I had to make to get up some of the climbs far out-stripped anything I remember having to put into my training prior to winning my World Masters' 5000m title in 1985 or training for and competing in any of the marathons that I was subsequently involved in.

The first ordeal, the ascent of the Devils Elbow, started barely half a dozen miles out of Blairgowrie at Bridge of Calley. Here, the A93 took a sharp right and began its relentless climb up to the Glenshee ski station, a haul of nearly 20 miles. It was a steady grind at first but on reaching Spittal of Glenshee, it upped the ante for the next 5-6 miles until just short of the summit where it spitefully cranked up the gradient to a degree that earn it the little arrows shown on the map.

In terms of length, this climb comes close to those found in the French Alps but, whereas the cols tend to meander their way up contours in order to ease gradients, the Scots, clearly can't be doing with such a waste of time and tarmac; they simply build their summit highways with a minimum of deviation. There is little more soul destroying on a bike than being able to see the next 20 - 30 minutes of your life stretching directly and inexorably ahead knowing that your physical distress is only going to intensify, especially if you have already engaged bottom gear.

We regrouped around the bus, which was waiting for us just over the summit and took on board a little sustenance in the form of fruit or energy bars. We also made some crucial adjustments to our clothing. For most of the lads this amounted to ensuring that they had sufficient protection against the scything, icy - cold airflow that they would encounter on the long, fast drop off the mountain.

Unfortunately, my problem was more intractable requiring a more radical solution. My hands were so wet and cold that I couldn't operate my gears or apply the brakes. This would rule me out of the descent if I didn't quickly get some feeling back into them. I removed the gloves and dried off my hands but then found that I couldn't get the gloves back on again, leaving me in an even worse predicament – no protection for my hands at all. I was very conscious that I had kept the other lads hanging around long enough in those grim conditions so there was only one solution: I would have to let Peter and

Steve take me in the bus down to Braemar to buy some effective gloves.

Away from the summit on the lower slopes of the mountain the conditions, although still very damp and gloomy, were far more tolerable and so I was soon able to rejoin the squad, resplendent in my new, chunky hand warmers. The detour meant that I missed about 20 miles of cycling.

All too soon our second major ascent to a ski station up in the clouds was upon us and, if anything, the road over the summit at Lecht was even tougher than Glenshee. It was desperately hard. I had to strain every bone and sinew to reach the top. It hurt. I was in considerable discomfort from my specific weaknesses – arm, back, shoulder, but also internally from the sheer strain of it all. I was exhausted; I was wet and I was cold and no, I wasn't enjoying it.

I am fairly sure the others felt much the same way so why were seven, otherwise reasonably well balanced adults subjecting themselves to such distress?

This is not an easy question to answer. I could say it is nothing more than the application of the "tight shoes" principle: you wear them simply to savour the blissful relief when you take them off! But, there is, of course, much more to it than that. It's about personal conditioning, parameter setting, proving your limits if you like or, in business-speak, "pushing the envelope". Even though an activity may appear extreme, masochistic or futile, the experience gained from it may well equip you to recognize and deal with other situations or events in your life however irrelevant the experience may at first appear. It seems to me that there are universal tenets, which can be applied to everything. There is also a powerful physiological component associated with sustained effort, namely, the release of endorphins, the body's natural anaesthetic. This can give a significant "high" and so I suppose we are no different to any other addict in that we are prepared to tolerate the unspeakable in order to obtain our fix. And, as with most addictions, the "high" can become increasingly difficult to satisfy.

The descent from Lecht summit was long and fast and only broken by the need to haul ourselves out of the glen at Bridge of Brown. This was another painfully steep climb but, mercifully, fairly short. We decided to look for some "later-than-usual" lunch in Grantown-on-Spey and were relieved to see the neon sign of a diner indicating that it was open for business. We were still cold and soggy despite the lick that we had maintained for the previous hour or so, but the ladies running the canteen-like establishment were very sympathetic towards our bedraggled state and served us up a lunch of soup, baguettes and cakes. They wished us well as we departed and even made a donation to the cause.

There were just 23 miles left to do and the road would be no worse than undulating; just a couple of little bumps to negotiate. What's more, the weather was visibly improving all the time so that this last, short, post-prandial hop into

Nairn, through a swathe of bright yellow broom, was a delightful way to end what had been a testing day.

By the time the day's grime had been pressure-washd from my various creases and crevices, Nairn was ablaze with evening sunshine, which I later felt I should have taken advantage of to explore the town. Once a flourishing fishing port, Nairn's sandy beaches and dunes had made it a popular holiday centre since Victorian times. On the face of it, therefore, it was somewhere well worth a nose around. Funnily enough, though, going for a walk was not at the forefront of my mind when I had just done 102 strenuous miles. Rather, my inclination on arriving at the digs was to crash out on the bed for an hour or so and give an astonishingly convincing impression of Ramases II. I imagined the others did much the same.

Transcript from audio-log
Where have you been?" "Dunno"
Although I approached this E2E journey as an athletic challenge rather than a sightseeing holiday it still seems like a missed opportunity to have absorbed so little of the places and landscape that we have ridden through. My recollections are largely just broad impressions. Worse still, there are stretches that I can't seem to recall at all. This is probably because a good deal of my attention is being directed into self-preservation in order to get through each day. This means making myself as energy efficient as possible. But minimizing energy loss and ensuring smooth delivery of effort requires considerable concentration. It's a game of numbers - pedal revolutions, heartbeats, intakes of breath;

each of which creates a rhythm that needs to be harnessed and harmonized for maximum efficiency - a bit like tuning a musical instrument. The greatest threat to this concentration in my experience is visual diversion (how often do we close our eyes to shut everything out when trying hard to compose ourselves or remember something?) Endurance athletes, in the main, can't do this because, of course, with the exception of some rowers, they usually like to see where they are going! Instead, they learn to block out all the ephemeral imagery by focusing on a point some distance in front of them, which has the effect of putting them in blinkers.

In my case, during the ride, whenever I need to muster all my reserves to overcome a rough patch, that point of focus is invariably the rear brake mechanism of whoever is riding immediately in front of me at the time. There have been quite a few of those rough patches, that much I do remember, which would go a long way towards explaining my lamentable recall of the trip (in the same way I had seen little of the surrounding countryside during the Marseilles – Cassis run 16 years earlier.) Peter, at least, makes the effort to acquaint himself with some of the stopover venues and other places of interest along the way and reaps the reward of some useful souvenir photos.

Fortunately, memories are rarely pure recollection of experience. They are more likely to be assemblages of many other things besides, for example, expectation, subsequently acquired information and a degree of creative primping or re-emphasis. I'm sure therefore, that in the fullness of time, I shall have all the stories I need about this momentous bike ride.

The rooming arrangements that we adopted in Sennen on our first night were, for the most part, maintained throughout the trip. Only Oz insisted on immediate change, which he expressed with a few of his more graphic 'bons mots' over breakfast that first morning. Having installed himself in a room containing 3 beds, he found he was sharing with a couple of dueling tubas. The intensity and duration of the pair's snoring had denied him, or so he claimed, even a wink of sleep. As there were 9 of us, a single occupancy room usually featured in our block reservation so the simple solution was to always let Oz have the odd room (shrewd one Oz.) Despite the virtuosity and gusto of the musical duo, remarkably they remained oblivious to each other's performance. Thankfully, therefore, the problem was immediately contained and, as far as I know, rooming then ceased to be an issue. Until we reached Nairn, that is, where the proprietor of the Guest House informed us he had several configurations of beds in rooms but not any twins. There followed a protracted interlude of misinterpretation and utter confusion as to how we could be accommodated but the upshot, as far as it related to me, was that Peter and I were still together but we were joined by 'Father Jack', John Mulvaney.

I had spent many a bleak mile riding in tandem with John over the previous week and it was his rear end, as often as not, that I locked onto when the going got particularly tough. His measured approach to the more extreme stretches of road drew me through many a crisis for which I shall remain eternally grateful. John is a veteran of many a successful cycling campaign both at home and abroad but, as he ably demonstrated near Ludlow and again in Altrincham, he does have a tendency to court misadventure. With a demeanor that nods in the direction of professorial, he seems to have developed the unfortunate knack of taking his eye off the ball at crucial moments so that, as well as periodically depositing skin on the highway, he has mastered the art of leaving vital equipment at home and abandoning good quality, and seemingly essential, items of clothing in wardrobes and bathrooms wherever he goes. With this in mind, I made a note to scour the room before leaving the next morning.

But Peter and I were not to be denied a little piece of vintage "Father Jack."

Transcript from audio-log
Whilst trying to dry out his gloves in our room, John drops one of them down the back of the radiator and then realises it can't be retrieved from the bottom because of the way the unit is boxed in. He decides the solution is to try and hook it out from the top with something suitably long and slender ... his pump. "Are you sure, John?" It only takes a few moments of dexterous waggling and a couple of determined thrusts and - voilà - that, too, becomes jammed behind the recalcitrant rad. John's face is a picture of disbelief and frustration and I have visions of things progressing inexorably, in Hoffnungesque fashion, to the eventual demolition of the whole house. John, of course, soon sees the funny side of his predicament and, we can only assume, found a way to retrieve his pump and liberate the capricious glove. Both are amongst his things now we've returned to the room after our meal, and the radiator, on the face of it at least, seems intact. I must remember to ask him how he did it.

Thursday 26th June

Nairn to Crask Inn (Highlands) Mileage 87m Ascent 4220ft

It was heartening to be setting off on the penultimate leg of our trip under an azure sky. The weather fronts that had been punishing us over the previous few days had suddenly and unexpectedly veered south leaving this north-eastern tip of Britain to enjoy a couple of much brighter, rain-free days. It was nice to have the sun shining as we busied ourselves loading up the bus, filling drinking bottles, stocking up with energy bars, pumping up tyres and debating whether the morning chill warranted the wearing of arm warmers: in other words, our morning routine. This morning, though, the atmosphere seemed different; it was lighter, looser than usual. Although there was still plenty of tough road ahead, it was a fact that the worst was now behind us and this realisation, together with the arrival of the sun, made us demob happy.

As we were putting the finishing touches to our preparations, a postman riding one of those red, single speed bikes with the cable operated drum brakes and big basket on the front for taking a hefty mailbag, rattled by with knees akimbo, insteps on pedals and feet at 10 to 2. By the size of his bag I guessed he had only just started out on his round. He looked over and kept his gaze on us until his head was at maximum swivel and he was on the verge of relinquishing control of his own destiny: then he was gone. But, just as we were about to mount up, he suddenly reappeared, pedaling furiously back in our direction. When he got level with us he looked worryingly distressed. I don't think he had exerted himself so much in a long time, if ever. It was a while before he was able to speak but it was worth the wait. In a lilt, which I couldn't begin to do justice to, he spluttered, "Ae saw ya sign on tha' van theer and I wanted tae help right enough but I didnae hae much cash, ya ken, and then I was awa doon th'road. But ae thought, aye, they should hae what aive got, right enough." He held out his hand and continued, "aim afraid it's oonly the 48 pence but that's all I have just noo."

That gesture probably denied him his subsidised canteen tea for the day. Lovely man. May all his mailbags be light ones.

Following that spiritually uplifting start to the day, we headed off towards the southwest and Inverness where we picked up the cycle path across Kessock Bridge. This spans the Moray Firth and is the principal route to and from Black Isle. Our first hour proved demanding as it was still fairly windy and we had been riding directly into it. However, just before the Bridge our road veered right and we were back on a predominantly northerly, wind-assisted tack once more.

The landscape was spectacular. Round every bend and atop every rise there was a fresh, broad vista on which to feast our eyes. We seemed to have it all now. The countryside immediately around us was rich and rolling much like it had been through the Borders. Up here, though, there were also vast tracts of water in the form of rivers, lochs and firths, which we constantly crossed, skirted or viewed from afar. And the mountains were by no means out of the frame; they were still there in the background. The panoramic view on the approach to the Cromarty Firth was one such vista that moved us sufficiently to stop for a photo shoot. Once across the bridge, we hugged the shoreline of the Firth until we reached Alness where we stopped for some lunch. I didn't take in much of Alness; all I recall is that one of the waitresses had, possibly, the most ample décolletage I had ever set eyes on and there was baked Alaska on the dessert menu. They made me smile in equal measure. The baked Alaska was quite something, too.

The awesome scenery continued long into the afternoon until we approached Lairg where it clouded over and the terrain began to turn into fairly featureless moorland. The last 15 miles or so up to the Crask Inn saw us entering one of Britain's true wildernesses where the only signs of civilisation were the peat workings along the roadside. We were pressing on now, heads down and eager to bring this stage to a close. I couldn't help feeling, though, that under different circumstances, the special beauty of the remote and seemingly barren countryside we were passing through would have mesmerized us all. As it was, our day had now begun to pall. Maybe this was a reaction to the "pointe sublime" overload we had experienced earlier in the day: but maybe we were all just shagged.

There was, however, one little ray of sunshine left waiting for us along this stretch of road; we had the pleasure and privilege of bumping into Rosie Swale Pope, the amazing lady who was running round the world on her own to raise awareness and funds for prostate cancer and a children's home in Russia. Her journey was scheduled to end in Tenby three months later. What an inspirational person: we had been duly humbled.

Splendid Isolation

When it eventually hove into view, the Crask Inn seemed eerily familiar – then the penny dropped; it was the "local shop for local people in Royston Vasey."[9]

Crask must be one of the remotest habitations in Britain located, as it is, at least a dozen miles from anywhere else in any direction. It comprises two buildings right on the roadside: the 19th century Inn itself where there is a bar, dining room and 3 en suite guest rooms and, 50m down the road, a cottage-type place that accommodates up to 10 people. From the outside this dwelling looks like an agricultural shed and outhouse surrounded by bog and

---

[9] Those familiar with the TV series " League of Gentlemen" will immediately be on message; everyone else must make do with my limp description of the place

assorted bucolic detritus. The inside is nowhere near as nice.

If you've ever been in a heavily used, poorly maintained, bottom of the range caravan then you will begin to get some idea of the interior and its furniture, fixtures and fittings. The showers and toilets looked unwelcoming and unsafe although, to be fair, they did prove more effective and comfortable than their initial appearance had suggested. Indeed, I found this to be the case with many aspects of the place. Being a veteran of many a night spent in mountain-side bothies and climbing huts, I have little trouble coming to terms with places like this and, as it happened, I had a particularly good night's sleep. There was no disputing, though, that the whole place was in desperate need of a major clean up. The kitchen area was especially rough and required nothing short of a good napalming. Oz put his finger on it when he suggested that, given all the entreaties issued by the Highland Council and other worthy bodies about protecting the Wildlands, a notice should be put up inside by the door requesting all users of the cottage to wipe their feet before leaving.

Thankfully, all the eating and drinking was done up at the inn and there were absolutely no complaints there. Nothing fancy, mind, just roasts and grills, puddings, pies and soups most of the ingredients of which were grown in the garden or on a nearby croft with the meat coming from local, hill-grazed livestock. Shame about the cottage but at £28.50 for bed, slap up breakfast and wholesome evening meal, we could hardly grumble.

After dinner we spent a very sociable evening in the bar with Mark and Debbie from Craven Arms, who were spending a few days gently pedaling in the area. They generously donated to the cause before the evening was out, which brought the amount of cash accumulated during the journey, from spontaneous donations like theirs', to over £100.

Meanwhile, the two on-line "Just Giving" funds, set up by Dangerous Dave and I, were continuing to receive donations, which we would discover when we got home, had amounted between them to some £14,000 before Gift Aid. It was a figure way beyond anything we ever expected to hand over to those dedicated, driven folk at The Cure Parkinson's Trust.

Friday 27th June

CRASK INN TO JOHN O' GROATS MILEAGE 81M ASCENT 3460FT

The final day dawns quietly save for the low level hubbub of what sounds like a truffle hunt taking place throughout the cottage. I have woken up far too early but I can't lie in, so perhaps I'll go and see what a wilderness is like off-peak. Outside, I look all around but focus on nothing. This isn't the first move in a scientifically developed "well-man" program that I'm about to launch into. No, it's because I've left my specs inside, which effectively means I can see nine tenths of Bugger All. But, never mind, the air is fresh and sweet and I don't need to see to breathe. I take a deep lungful and hold onto it, after which I experience a heady moment of complete calm. This intrigues me and, not being overburdened with things to do at this point, I decide to work on it to see how far down the road to Nirvana I can get. There is little to distract me visually, as I've explained, and there are moments of complete silence when the breeze drops. "Touch" I can eliminate by standing like George W Bush, arms slightly away from my sides, and thinking myself down by means of a relaxation sequence I learnt somewhere. That just leaves "smell" and "taste" but the Parkinson's relieved me of those two conspirators many years ago. So, picture this. Here I am, devoid of all my senses, poised like a B-Movie gunslinger, clad in just tee shirt, under-pants and loafers, and standing in the middle of a national highway trying to create enough good karma to take me to Nirvana.

The things you'll do when you think nobody is looking, eh?

My return to sanity was abrupt when I realised that I had fallen victim to the thing I'd feared most since entering more northerly latitudes. My lower legs and feet appeared to be shrouded in mist, only it wasn't mist but a dense swarm of midges. I shot back inside as quickly as I could without creating a disturbance and applied liberal amounts of "After Midge." But, too late: they'd had a field day. At least my experience would enable me to remind the others. With all that stagnant water around the place we were slap in the middle of Midge Mecca. I went back to bed and waited for the itching to start.

By the time we got going a wind had got up that promised to blow us all the way to the end of the British mainland. We quickly settled into a very respectable pace, which we maintained for a good couple of hours. We sped through Strath Bagastie and on to Altnaharra where we turned off onto the B873, which ran all the way to Bettyhill on the north-facing coast of Britain. It was a magnificent road for cycling; it gently undulated through the full length of Strath Naver first along the edge of Loch Naver then skirting the banks of the River of the same name. The strath was wide and open offering a big sky yet the mountains still flanked us in the distance. We were making great time - 20 miles were clocked in the hour and, boy, did I love this!

As we were going so well we decided to keep going and get in as many miles as possible before lunch. Bettyhill came and went at about the 35-mile mark. The average speed was still over 17mph. But that was about to change.

The previous day I had started to feel profoundly tired towards the middle of the afternoon but today it occurred much earlier, which was, presumably, the additional price I had to pay for having the audacity to mix it with the others in the charge up Strath Naver. We were now on the A836, Britain's most northerly A road that runs west-east along the flat top of the mainland. It affords fine views of the Atlantic coastline but, in contrast to the terrain we had been enjoying earlier, it proved to be a serious roller coaster that was constantly descending into bays and then rising steeply back out again. I started to find the climbs just a little too long and the descents just a little too short and it wasn't long before I was really struggling and having to dig deep to find the strength and willpower to keep going. "Le velo c'est la souffrance" is a popular French adage that, during my worst moments, I kept repeating to myself. I found this helped providing I alternated it with an old British cry along the lines of, "Sod the French" although what I actually said was more alliterative.

Our final lunch stop was at the Park Hotel in Thurso: what a lifesaver! The bar met all our sustenance needs in pleasant surroundings and even offered some pudding favourites for good measure. (Yes, of course I did).

Happy in the knowledge we were all going to make it in together, we set off on the final, short and relatively gentle stretch of the A836 - just 20 miles or so - into

John O'Groats. The sun was shining brightly just as it had been when we departed from Lands End. How symmetrical!

They say that the most frequently heard utterance in J O'G is, "where to next?" And it's true; it really is almost impossible not to say it when you get there. But this is not because you are immediately inspired by the place to start planning your next major odyssey or display of intrepidity, but simply that this one-eyed little hamlet with the allure of a Canvey Island caravan site, is such an anti-climax. I concluded that "where to next?" must really mean, "let's get the hell outta this godforsaken place".

After a repeat performance of the photography antics we went through prior to leaving Land's End, we made our way swiftly back up the road to our hotel for the night and lost no time acquainting ourselves with the bar where we met other equally jubilant end to enders who all had stories to tell.

The most vocal and jocular amongst them were two firemen who had cycled up from the West Midlands. They had clearly arrived well before us and appeared not to have wasted a moment in starting the process of anaesthetizing themselves for the night ahead under canvas. They had been on the road for three weeks and were traveling heavy. They had everything you could imagine piled up on their bikes including fishing tackle. I've rarely seen two bikes more laden. I tried to lift one; I didn't even get the front wheel off the ground. I would have bet good money that there was a porcelain sink in one of the front panniers. But apart from their incredible weight the other remarkable thing about the two bikes was their state of disrepair. They were ill fitting, low specification, mountain bikes to begin with, which alone must have made life in the saddle a chore for the two riders, but it was also obvious that neither of the machines had ever received any maintenance. The rear gear cogs were dry and worn to sharp points and the chains made the one taken off Jezzer's bike a few days before look good for another couple of years.

It was a miracle the guys had made it as far as they had. We decided against any closer inspection. The two lads claimed they had spent £6 on accommodation, presumably campsite fees incurred when their opportunism and resourcefulness ran out one night. As a rule they would just pitch their tents more or less wherever they felt like it and I got the distinct impression that they wouldn't be giving that any thought until chucking out time. These boys were made of tough stuff but were as genial a duo as you could wish to meet. Brave or barmy? Either way I couldn't help but admire their spirit especially when they admitted they rarely ever rode bikes, but were simply a couple of regular work chums who had decided to "just ... do it for the Firefighters Benevolent Fund!" For the second time in as many days, we felt humbled by the exploits of fellow travelers.

If we'd had to ride their bikes could we have "just ... done it"? None of us relished the thought but we agreed it would be do-able – eventually. Ethnic Australians have their 'laws of least effort' to enable them to survive the heat of the day and one of their edicts says, "You can achieve anything you like so long as you are not in a hurry". Maybe so, but attempting such a journey equipped like that, even if given all the time in the world, would mean missing out on THE vital component of the whole exercise - the euphoria of riding fluently on a good bike. If I could bottle that sensation I would become a major contributor towards universal health and happiness overnight. But, as you will have gathered by now the stuff doesn't come cheap but requires sound investment particularly during the development stages in order to achieve the optimum yield.

As the conclusion of our odyssey fell a day short of the umpteenth anniversary of the birth of one, David "Oz" Osborn, our evening meal celebrated both auspicious occasions. The juxtaposition of the two dates also started me wondering how the pain of my labours up Lecht and the Devil's Elbow compared to those suffered by Mrs Osborn when delivering baby David into this world all those eons ago. (*Yes, yes, I know, but I'd had a hard day*)

The meal provided me with one last little treat; it introduced me to clootie dumpling. Not generally found south of the border, it was a dessert that appeared to be a cross between bread and butter pudding, bread pudding and Christmas cake and had the consistency of a medicine ball. Top tuck all the same, especially with a side of hot, creamy custard.

After dinner we reinstalled ourselves in the bar and carried on supping until we started to fall victim to fatigue and emotion. This led to a string of expansive "goodnights", excessive apologies for early departure and effusive "farewells" all round, as each of us in turn lurched and stumbled our way up to bed. At least, that's how I progressed to my room, but then that is how I usually move around these days.

We left our firemen friends to it, seemingly, still in full swing. They evidently felt they needed a general rather than a local anaesthetic to get them through the night. The following morning there was no sign of the two lads and the bikes were gone from where they had been parked at the side of the hotel. All that remained were four deep indentations in the asphalt where the wheels had been: a fitting testimony to endeavour, determination, resilience and crap bikes.

Aftermath

Over the years I've had a recurring dream in which I am coaching a group of promising runners. As I impart my advice to the athletes I find myself joining in and running fluently and effortlessly alongside them: I am at the top of my game. Then I wake up and the disappointment on realizing it was all a dream is profound.

Those 12 days in the saddle in the summer of 2008 offered many similar, sublime moments only, unlike my dream, they were wonderfully real: they did not disappoint and I ultimately prevailed over a true challenge: not one that was "good for my age": not one that was "good, given my circumstances" but an achievement in absolute terms – "my bloody terms!"

We rode 1030 miles and climbed over 63,000ft at an average speed of 15 mph. I would have been pleased with those statistics 40 years ago but to achieve them at this stage of the game was especially gratifying. By demonstrating that I had regained the ability to ride more or less all day over distances in excess of 100 miles, I had, effectively, turned my clock back decades and rediscovered my cycling horizons of old. Rides I had assumed were way beyond my capability had become accessible again; the future will be so much richer now. The ride also showed, to my satisfaction at least, that muscles affected by Parkinson's can be trained up and their function improved. Far from causing distress for me and distraction for the group, my Parkinson's rarely imposed itself while I was riding, which has since led me to conclude that what principally governed how I performed on the bike had little or nothing to do with PD but was simply how athletically fit I was: how many quality miles I had under my belt and how I utilized past experience – just as it always used to be.

Unsteadiness on my feet, dyskynesia[10], freezing[11] and sometimes tremor, or any permutation of the above, would usually emerge to some extent an hour or so after reaching our destination each day. This was fine by me although it couldn't have made me very good company in the evenings. Then again, perhaps it didn't notice much as we all hit our beds fairly early. This patterning did surprise me, however, because even calm, relaxed days at home were rarely as consistently symptom-free as this. It got me thinking about what was going on here and, despite an absence of anything even vaguely scientific by way of evidence, or much inclination to dwell on it over long, I came up wih a theory regarding my condition. It was this.

My Parkinson's is basically a weak, cowardly force that struggles to thrive in a positive, controlled, high-energy environment. Its perniciousness lies in its effectiveness as an infinitely patient opportunist that bides its time until, inevitably, I am obliged, for one reason or another, to reduce my energy level to one it can tolerate at which time it re-asserts its influence and starts inflicting on me its dubious sense of humour.

---

[10] Dyskynesia: involuntary movement
[11] Freezing: difficulty in initiating/maintaining movement

More seriously, I have learnt not to be deterred too readily from doing, or at least exploring, seemingly difficult or demanding activity on the grounds that the Parkinson's won't allow it. The perversity of Parkinson's is such that something that is hard in the commonly held order of things may, in the event, prove easier than something deemed mundane; for example, I would fare far better hiking 20 miles over rough terrain than pack and pay for just a few items at a busy supermarket check-out.

Our pedal-powered potter up the deck, from bow to stern, of the good ship Great Britain, has now been consigned to Old Portlian folklore, but I sense the bigger voyage I am on has still to reach open waters. So, what's next? (You see, the spirit of John O' Groats gets you in the end!) In terms of cycling, there remains one major ride out there, which goads me and which I fear I may get drawn into eventually, "La Marmotte." This route is 174 km long in the French Alps and features more than 5180 metres of climbing. The event, which takes place at the end of June, goes over the Col du Glandon, Col du Telegraphe, Col du Galibier and finishes at the top of one the most famous Tour de France climbs, L' Alpe d'Huez. I've driven all the roads on many occasions and ridden parts of the route at odd times over the years and I wouldn't argue for a moment with its claim to be the toughest single-day amateur ride in the world. A quest too far for me? Yes, it probably would be especially if it turns out blisteringly hot as it frequently does. We shall have to see.

Of course, not all challenges are picked and chosen. I have already embarked on my next challenge and it doesn't involve the bike or any sport. Some time ago my speech started to become an effort and my delivery got softer and less distinct to a point where my ability to communicate properly was becoming compromised: my voice projection had the impact of a duck fart on a muggy day. It was time to broach the subject with my consultant who arranged for me to go through an intensive 4-week "Lee Silverman Voice Treatment" programme. This entailed rigorous training of the vocal chords on a daily basis, which I will need to continue for myself if a significant and lasting change is to be achieved. But that shouldn't be a problem: I shall simply bring to it the same principles and disciplines that I have applied to bike riding and running. The sessions were what I always imagined singing lessons to be like. If that is the case, then maybe I'll be able to sing in due course. Now that really would be something: I've always wanted to be able to sing. Perhaps this will turn out to be a challenge of choice, after all.

One further oddity emerged after we got back home from LeJOG. All those who did the ride lost weight – except me. I put on 4 kilos – over half a stone.

I can't begin to imagine what could have caused that!

Appendix 1

The Bike

Frame	De Rosa "King X-Light" full carbon
Chainset	Campagnolo Record 50x34
Brakes	Campagnolo Record Titanium
Rear Mech	Campagnolo Record Titanium 10 speed
Front Mech	Campagnolo Record Titanium
Cassette	Campagnolo Record 13 - 26
Wheels	Fulcrum Racing 1
Tyres	Michelin Pro 2
Tubes	Michelin Latex
Saddle	Fizik Aliante carbon
Pedals	Time RXS
Stem	Time carbon
Bars	Reynolds Ouzo Pro
Weight	**16.5lbs**

Appendix 2

The Medication

Time	Sinemet Plus – 125 mg	Sinemet LS 62.5mg	Amantadine 100mg	Entacapone 200mg	Rotigotine Patches 2x4mg
7.00	2	-	1	1	1
8.30	1	-	-	-	
10.00	-	1	-	1	
11.30	1	-	-	-	
13.00	-	1	1	1	
14.30	1	-	-	-	
16.00	1	-	1	1	
17.30	1	-	-	-	
19.00	-	1	-	1	
20.30	1	-	-	-	
22.00	-	1	-	1	
Total	8	4	3	6	

This "little and often" regime is the result of careful self-assessment and titration over the past 16 years. Starting with 3 x Sinemet 62.5 per day in July 1993 I subsequently made over 30 adjustments as the PD progressed - usually small additions (except when a new drug proved effective and was added e.g. Entacapone in November 2001 and Amantadine in July 2006, when I was able to reduce the daily dosage of Sinemet.) Each change usually involved a short period of trial and error to ensure I was achieving the minimum effective dosage.

I went straight onto Sinemet within a few months of being diagnosed. My original consultant was of the school that questioned the virtue of forgoing the most effective treatment in order to delay possible, but not inevitable, complications at some time in the future. I can only say that I think his strategy has worked for me so far.

Popping pills every hour and a half is not without its difficulties especially on a bike! However, these have been largely overcome with the aid of specially modified pill boxes and a sports watch with a facility called "countdown repeat". It can be set to sound an alarm at the end of whatever period is required in perpetuity; in my case every 90 minutes. Such watches can be found in both the Timex and Casio ranges.

Lightning Source UK Ltd.
Milton Keynes UK
24 August 2009
143021UK00001B/4/P